"This comprehensive guide takes a compassiona Intuitive Eating for diabetes. Clear and practica reflects on emotional health, and empowers readers to develop a sustainable relationship with food. An invaluable resource for anyone with diabetes seeking to heal body and mind using Intuitive Eating."

—**Erin Phillips, MPH, RD, CDCES**, weight-inclusive diabetes dietitian, and host of the *Glucose Riot* podcast

"As an internist who specializes in eating disorders, I read Janice Dada's book with joy. It is practical, compassionate, scientifically sound, and beautifully presented, with case presentations that make her teachings come to life. I will be recommending this regularly to my patients, because THIS is what the standard of care should be!"

—**Jennifer L. Gaudiani, MD, CEDS-C, FAED**, founder and medical director of the Gaudiani Clinic, and author of *Sick Enough*

"This book provides a comprehensive toolkit for whole-person diabetes care. Managing diabetes is a daily commitment; having a playbook to support both mental and physical well-being is essential."

—**Gregory Dodell, MD**, Central Park Endocrinology

"*Intuitive Eating for Diabetes* offers a compassionate, science-based approach to diabetes care, blending Intuitive Eating principles with blood sugar management. This transformative guide shifts away from the weight-centric model, providing practical tools to reconnect with your body and honor your health. Essential for individuals navigating diabetes or prediabetes—and for professionals seeking to deliver inclusive, empowering care—it redefines diabetes management with practical tools to make sustainable changes."

—**Wendy Lopez, MS, RD, CDCES**, cofounder of Diabetes Digital and Food Heaven

"For a long time, there has been a need for a resource that helps individuals manage their diabetes while maintaining their quality of life and enjoying food. This book is finally the solution!"

—**Sumner Brooks, MPH, RDN**, coauthor of *How to Raise an Intuitive Eater*

"In this much-needed resource, Janice Dada offers a clear path to manage diabetes without blame, shame, and food deprivation. Instead, *Intuitive Eating for Diabetes* will show you how to let go of the diet mindset, understand your body's needs, and help you learn to care for yourself in a way that supports your physical and emotional well-being without a focus on weight loss. Read this book, and then pass it on to others who will also benefit from the wisdom contained in these pages!"

—**Judith Matz, LCSW**, coauthor of *The Emotional Eating, Chronic Dieting, Binge Eating, and Body Image Workbook* and *Beyond a Shadow of a Diet*

"This book is a breath of fresh air for people with diabetes who have been bound to restrictive, one-size-fits-all approaches to food. Dada's perspective—based on the latest empirical research and two decades of clinical experience—is accessible, personalized, and comprehensive. She masterfully demystifies diabetes management, explaining everything from understanding your diagnosis to interpreting labs to self-advocacy with health care providers. This is an essential, one-of-a-kind resource!"

—**Erin D. Basinger**, associate professor of communication studies at University of North Carolina at Charlotte

"Finally, a book I can share with my clients who are looking for non-diet support to manage diabetes! With *Intuitive Eating for Diabetes*, Janice shows readers that they can care for their health without turning to restrictive, unsustainable diet plans. It takes the shame and fear out of a diagnosis and replaces it with realistic, evidence-based advice for navigating life with diabetes."

—**Rachael Hartley, RD**, author of *Gentle Nutrition*

"In a world where weight loss and fear dominate the messaging about diabetes, Janice provides a valuable alternative path. This book is an essential resource for building knowledge about diabetes and for managing this condition using a kinder, more compassionate, and weight-inclusive approach."

—**Aaron Flores, RDN**, registered dietitian nutritionist, certified Body Trust specialist, and host of the *Men Unscripted* podcast

INTUITIVE EATING

FOR
DIABETES

The **No Shame, No Blame, Non-Diet Approach** *to* Managing Your Blood Sugar

JANICE DADA, MPH, RDN

New Harbinger Publications, Inc.

Publisher's Note

This publication is designed to provide accurate and authoritative information in regard to the subject matter covered. It is sold with the understanding that the publisher is not engaged in rendering psychological, financial, legal, or other professional services. If expert assistance or counseling is needed, the services of a competent professional should be sought.

NEW HARBINGER PUBLICATIONS is a registered trademark of New Harbinger Publications, Inc.

New Harbinger Publications is an employee-owned company.

The Intuitive Eating Scale 3 is reproduced from Tylka, T. L., C. Maïano, M. Fuller-Tyszkiewicz, J. Linardon, C. B. Burnette, J. Todd, and V. Swami. 2024. "The Intuitive Eating Scale-3: Development and psychometric evaluation." *Appetite* 199: 107407. Reprinted by permission of Elsevier.

Cover design by Amy Shoup; Acquired by Ryan Buresh; Edited by Rebecca Job

---

Library of Congress Cataloging-in-Publication Data on file

Printed in the United States of America

27   26   25
10   9   8   7   6   5   4   3   2   1   First Printing

To those living with diabetes.
May you find peace with food and your body.

Contents

Foreword

As the coauthor of *Intuitive Eating*, I was honored when Janice Dada, the author of this remarkable book, asked me to write the foreword. I was also grateful to have the privilege and opportunity to help bring this healing approach into the world of diabetes treatment.

Within moments of being diagnosed with diabetes, you'll likely find yourself in a cloud of uncertainty. You might ask, "What am I going to do? How do I manage this? How do I eat?" In the traditional care of diabetes, treatment is offered as a set of rules, leading to the fear that life the way you know it has suddenly been taken away from you. There might be feelings of shame and responsibility for "getting diabetes" and anger that this is happening to you.

Unfortunately, we live in a weight-centric world, which is driven by diet culture. This can influence traditional diabetes treatment—treatment that is typically focused on weight loss. After the initial period of attempting to follow the rules perfectly, such as "lose weight" and "don't eat many carbs," many people find these strictures unsustainable, and they blame and shame themselves even more. A painful sense of deprivation and an underlying rebellion can set in—a force that goes against their innate desire for self-care and determination to be the best patient.

This sense of rebellion is a natural outcome of our need to assert autonomy, despite its consequences. Toddlers and teenagers regularly deal with these rebellious feelings. And for each adult who has developed a healthy ego, there is an inner toddler/teen evoked by any external rules they are expected to follow.

Intuitive Eating for Diabetes offers an alternative way of approaching diabetes care. A way that respects your autonomy, reconnecting you to your internal wisdom about eating. As a result, you'll feel an openness emerging to taking in guidelines drawn for self-care, self-compassion, and sustainability—none of which brings a negative reaction to the treatment. The pathway to this self-care is drawn by working on the four pillars of intuitive eating for diabetes. Each pillar is built on a foundation of scientific research and practical advice, offering the intuitive eating framework as a route toward blood sugar improvement.

Before learning about the four pillars, each person, whether newly diagnosed with diabetes or managing it for many years, must challenge a very basic but misguided myth that someone with diabetes must lose weight to keep their blood sugar under control. Both the medical community and the lay public have been influenced by diet culture promoting the belief that anything that ails one will be fixed by losing weight. Unfortunately, this pervasive belief does not consider the well-established fact that no sustainable method for intentional weight loss exists. In fact, any attempt at weight loss raises the risk of weight cycling, as one goes through the rigors of restriction to the rebound of weight gain. Over and over and over! Weight cycling—losing and gaining the same or more weight—has been shown to be pro-inflammatory and might cause fluctuations in cardiovascular risk factors, such as blood pressure and heart rate. It has also been shown to increase one's risk of developing type 2 diabetes (T2DM). Ironic, isn't it, that the prevailing notion that someone diagnosed with T2DM must lose weight to control their blood sugar, while this repeatedly unsuccessful pursuit might actually increase their risk!

Several research studies have supported the value of using the principles of intuitive eating in managing blood sugar for people with diabetes. One study that looked at people with T2DM who were not on insulin found that intuitive eating was associated with an 89 percent lower chance of having poor glycemic control, while another found increased body satisfaction. Others have shown lower blood pressure and triglycerides.

And if you're still dubious and scared, reading anecdotes that describe the lived experience of those who have been tainted by diet culture, rejected it, and found improved diabetes management will help you feel not so alone on your journey.

Now, let's take a brief look at the four pillars of intuitive eating for diabetes. The first and foremost pillar involves challenging diet culture by creating a diet-free mindset. Although this challenge goes against everything that has been taught about treating diabetes, you must leave behind the futility and dangers of diet culture and embrace a way that can lead you to the freedom that comes with trusting your internal wisdom about eating.

The next three pillars address diabetes self-care, gentle nutrition, and your individualized treatment plan—all of which focus on self-compassion, self-care, and mindful awareness. Here you will find the tools to reclaim your intuitive eating wisdom. Showing kindness and respect toward your body while learning to find satisfaction in your eating will lower your stress and bring you to a place of body attunement, inner peace, and safety.

—Elyse Resch, MS, RDN, CEDS-S, FAND

Nutrition therapist
Coauthor of *Intuitive Eating, The Intuitive Eating Workbook,* and *The Intuitive Eating Card Deck*
Author of *The Intuitive Eating Workbook for Teens* and *The Intuitive Eating Journal*

Introduction

Several years ago, a client with diabetes whom I'd been working with for some time asked me how I got interested in diabetes as a person who doesn't actually have the condition. Her question got me thinking: *Why am I so passionate about diabetes care and education?* I thought back to the people I'd known and worked with who had diabetes over the years. First to mind was my own family history with diabetes. My late grandfather had type 2 diabetes at a time when diabetes management and education was still in its infancy. While I was too young to understand what was happening at the time, I'm told my grandfather was determined to manage his blood sugar without medications. Unfortunately, this choice didn't serve his situation well and he eventually suffered consequences from that decision. In addition, my mom had gestational diabetes while pregnant with me. For my mom, there wasn't the scrupulous monitoring that today's women with GDM tend to have, and consequently, her delivery had a nearly tragic outcome. Thankfully, diabetes care has come such a long way since then!

I also considered my education and training—for instance, how as a dietetic intern I was instructed to use a standard one-size-fits-all reduced-carbohydrate meal plan for those with diabetes, regardless of the person's size, appetite, or physical activity level. Those meal plans were such an unrealistic match for most patients! In addition, I thought of my clients in larger bodies who were given impossible directives to eat tiny portions, lose weight by any means, undergo irreversible surgeries, take medications with debilitating side effects, and exercise through pain and disability if they wanted a shot at improving their diabetes outcomes. Even as an inexperienced intern, I knew there had to be a better way.

During the course of my nearly two-decade career as a registered dietitian and diabetes educator, I've worked with countless individuals who've suffered because of diet culture's influence over diabetes recommendations. I've had clients take diabetes management way too far, developing eating disorders as a result, and others who threw in the towel because it all seemed impossible. *Intuitive Eating for Diabetes* is here to change the diabetes self-management landscape by bringing together a weight-inclusive eating framework built on self-compassion and body attunement with the science of blood sugar management. *Intuitive Eating for Diabetes* is the first book of its kind to formally apply the principles of intuitive eating to a medical condition. *Intuitive eating* is a way of eating that is directed by a mind-body connection integrating instinct, emotion, and rational thought (Tribole and Resch 2020). Registered dietitians Evelyn Tribole and Elyse Resch first fearlessly pioneered this concept back in the 1990s. Today, there are over two hundred scientific studies highlighting the benefits of intuitive eating, which include increased well-being, lower risk of eating disorders, and improved metabolic markers. Research supports the use of an intuitive eating framework as a valuable tool for blood sugar improvement (Pires Soares et al. 2021; Wheeler et al. 2016; Willig et al. 2014)!

The ten principles of intuitive eating can steer those with or at risk for diabetes toward intrinsic eating based on internal cues, away from dieting and external rules that almost always backfire, and toward positive self-care. Tylka et al. (2019) found intuitive eating to be associated with greater weight stability, which is critical given that weight cycling is a risk factor for negative medical, metabolic, and psychological health outcomes (O'Hara and Taylor 2018). The weight-centric health care model for diabetes clearly isn't working—more people than ever have diabetes, and research repeatedly shows that diets cause harm. It's time for diabetes care to be delivered without blame, shame, and stigma. Applying the principles of intuitive eating to diabetes does just this; it allows for the focus to move from weight to actual health-promoting behaviors.

Getting the Most Out of This Book

I sure love to relax with a book at the end of the day, but this isn't the type of book you'll want to read in bed at night. If you're sleepy or distracted while reading, you may miss some important information. I'd suggest setting aside a certain number of minutes each day or week in which you'll plan to read and reflect. I find this often works best if you connect it with another activity that you always do. For example, if you sit down and drink coffee or tea at the table every morning, keep your book next to your favorite mug as a reminder to spend ten minutes reading each day. If you do this, you'll have read for more than an hour by the end of the week!

Throughout the book, you'll notice headings titled "Reflection," where you'll be invited to reflect on your personal experience with the topic just discussed. Try not to skip over these, as they do offer you an important opportunity to apply what you've read to your own circumstance. Also, I'd recommend using a dedicated journal or notebook for these activities so that all of your notes are together (I'll refer to this as your companion journal throughout).

There are many case examples throughout the book that you may find relatable. Keep in mind that you should always discuss any changes to your own personal diabetes management with your medical team. The cases I highlight are only meant as examples, not as suggestions. Also, with the exception of chapter 9, the case examples throughout the book are amalgams of various clients I've worked with over the years. Names and details have been changed for privacy. However, in chapter 9 you'll have the opportunity to read about three individuals I worked with who graciously offered to personally share their experiences with you.

Lastly, please be kind and gentle with yourself as you read through this book. There are no expectations for how quickly you move through it, and there is no "success" or "failure" in this process. Intuitive eating is all about discovering your unique needs and that will take time, curiosity, and exploration. I'm so glad you're here!

CHAPTER 1

Diabetes, Explained

If you've been told you have diabetes or prediabetes, then you have something in common with 135.7 million Americans—nearly half of the entire US population! As of 2021, 38.1 million US adults had diabetes, and 97.6 million had prediabetes (CDC 2024). But diabetes' impact extends far beyond the US: around the globe, diabetes affects approximately 537 million adults. A slowdown in diabetes rates isn't expected anytime soon; in fact, rates are expected to continue rising around the world (IDF [International Diabetes Federation] 2021).

Research and the lived experiences of people with diabetes (like you!) has added to our knowledge base and understanding of this condition in tremendous ways over time. Can you believe it was only about a hundred years ago that insulin was first discovered? In the pages that follow, you'll learn things you're probably not hearing in the doctor's office or the popular media. You may feel emotions ranging from relief to anger after reading what I'm about to present. My own clients have asked me in frustration why they aren't hearing this information from other health care providers. My hope is that readers like you will be able to use this book as a resource for your own personal care and self-advocacy.

As you've likely experienced firsthand, health professionals often place an immense focus on restrictive diets and weight management to treat diabetes. Given that diabetes cases are rising steadily, it's clear this weight-centric approach isn't working. For this reason, you won't find any weight loss directives or food restrictions here. Instead, we'll shift the focus to health-promoting behaviors.

In this first chapter, you'll learn about diabetes types, diagnosis, and the root causes of diabetes development. We'll take a deep dive into weight science and the harms of dieting, including the problematic history of weight classifications. In addition, we'll address weight bias and self-advocacy strategies. You'll learn how a focus on health-promoting behaviors rather than body weight can positively impact your diabetes. This chapter will give you a better understanding of diabetes and an enthusiasm for learning a new, non-diet, self-compassionate way to manage this condition. Let's dive in!

What Is Diabetes?

Let's start with some basics. As you likely already know, diabetes is a health condition in which the body has trouble turning food into energy. Typically, when you eat foods containing carbohydrates, the digestive process will break carbohydrates down into individual glucose (sugar) molecules, which provides cells with vital food energy they need. The glucose enters your bloodstream and triggers your pancreas to release a hormone called insulin. Insulin helps move glucose into cells so the glucose can provide energy for metabolic processes. With diabetes, the body is either resistant to the insulin being released or there isn't enough insulin being produced to help get glucose into the cells. This means your cells don't get the vital food energy they need and glucose accumulates in the bloodstream.

To further comprehend what's happening in your body, imagine that each cell surface has a lock and the insulin is the key to open the lock (see figure 1). With type 2 diabetes, it's as if the insulin-resistant cells have changed the lock and insulin doesn't have the new key. This means the pancreas is sending out insulin, but the cell is ignoring it! Because of this, glucose piles up in the bloodstream outside the cell. Triggered by the elevated glucose, the pancreas sends out even more insulin to try and get glucose into the cells.

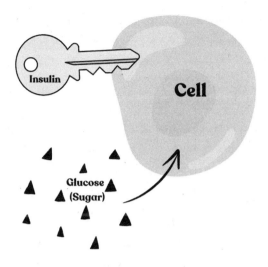

Figure 1

Since insulin is a fat storage hormone and the insulin-resistant body has high levels of insulin being sent out by the pancreas, weight gain is likely a *symptom* of T2DM and insulin resistance rather than simply the cause. In other words, when insulin resistance is present, the pancreas will just keep pumping out more insulin. The more insulin there is in circulation, the more weight the body is likely to gain. Considering this, isn't it odd that doctors routinely tell people with insulin resistance to lose weight as if it's so easy to do?

Your body tries its best to remove excess glucose from the bloodstream by eliminating it in the urine. Thus, high blood glucose leads to frequent urination (polyuria), increased thirst (polydipsia), and the incomplete digestion and absorption of food energy leads to increased hunger (polyphagia). If you've ever experienced this phenomenon, you know it may feel like you are starving—because metabolically speaking, your cells *are* starving! In addition, when there is extra glucose in the bloodstream, this increases the viscosity of the blood. Thick, sugary blood can lead to macrovascular problems (relating to large blood vessels, like arteries) and microvascular problems (affecting our smallest blood vessels, like those in the eyes and kidneys), such as blurry vision and eventual microvascular eye damage, poorly healing wounds, kidney issues, neuropathy, and cardiovascular problems.

Types of Diabetes

There are many types of diabetes and many ways to diagnose the condition. You likely already know the type of diabetes you have. The types of diabetes and the typical treatments that are offered for each, follow (ADA [American Diabetes Association] 2023):

- **Type 1 diabetes mellitus (T1DM):** This is an autoimmune condition—when the immune system attacks its own healthy tissue, organs, or cells—that results in complete insulin deficiency. It represents 5 to 10 percent of all diabetes cases.

  Treatment: Insulin

- **Type 2 diabetes mellitus (T2DM):** This is a non-autoimmune condition that leads to progressive loss of adequate insulin secretion and is related to genetics, inflammation, and metabolic stress. It represents 90 to 95 percent of all diabetes cases.

  Treatment: Oral medication, injectable medication, insulin, and/or lifestyle changes

- **Gestational diabetes mellitus (GDM):** This is diabetes that is diagnosed in the second or third trimester of pregnancy. It's a temporary diabetes as a result of insulin resistance in pregnancy.

  Treatment: Oral medication, insulin, and/or lifestyle changes

- **Latent autoimmune diabetes in adults (LADA):** This is an incomplete, slowly developing form of T1DM with mild to moderate insulin resistance. It's also called diabetes type 1.5.

  Treatment: Insulin, and in early stages, possibly oral or injectable medications

- **Secondary diabetes:** This is a form of insulin-dependent diabetes that isn't autoimmune in nature. Potential causes include accident or injury to the pancreas, pancreatitis, cystic fibrosis, substance abuse, steroid use, cancer or HIV/AIDS treatment, post-organ transplant, and infection.

  Treatment: Oral medication, insulin, attention to the underlying cause

- **Other forms of diabetes:** This includes neonatal diabetes and maturity-onset diabetes of the young (MODY).

  Treatment: Oral medication, injectable medication, insulin, and/or lifestyle changes

DIAGNOSING DIABETES

If you've already been diagnosed with diabetes, then you likely know some of the options for blood testing. If not, here's what you should know: diabetes can be diagnosed four different ways: a fasting blood glucose test, an oral glucose tolerance test, a hemoglobin A1c test (HbA1c), or a random, non-fasting blood glucose test. The American Diabetes Association (ADA) has cutoff criteria for all of these tests for both diabetes and prediabetes.

There's also a condition known as *prediabetes*, in which blood sugar levels are higher than they "should" be, but not yet high enough to qualify for a diabetes diagnosis.

Prediabetes

There's some controversy around this diagnosis. According to investigative journalist Charles Piller, the term resulted from a brainstorming session of six diabetes thought leaders hoping to elevate the level of concern in patients and doctors for a high blood sugar that was not quite diabetes (Piller 2019). Despite other specialists in the field citing weak support and even scaremonger-ing, the ADA and Centers for Disease Control and Prevention (CDC) went on to declare prediabetes as the first step on the path to diabetes.

To this day, the World Health Organization (WHO) and other medical authorities remain unconvinced that prediabetes rou-tinely leads to diabetes or that existing treatments do much good, rejecting the idea of a prediabetes diagnostic category altogether. And it makes sense: a 2018 comprehensive review of 103 studies showed that most people in the prediabetes range never actually progressed to diabetes over any period studied. In fact, 59 percent of the prediabetes patients studied returned to normal blood glucose values in one to eleven years without any treatment (Richter et al. 2018)!

Still, the diagnosis of prediabetes remains common. Piller points out how the realities of the medical establishment and its financial ties, particularly in the US, complicate matters even further. There is no Food and Drug Administration (FDA) approved treatment for prediabetes, so many clinicians prescribe diabetes medications "off label" that carry the risk of side effects. The American College of Physicians has rated the ADA's financial con-flicts with drug companies as among the most extreme. In fact, seven of the fourteen ADA experts who wrote the 2018 standards of care for prediabetes received between $41,000 and $6.8 million from diabetes drug and device companies between 2013 and 2017 (Piller 2019).

In this sense, the controversy around prediabetes reveals some of the problems with the way diabetes is currently treated and dis-cussed—problems you've likely encountered in your treatment journey. If most people with elevated blood sugar are never actu-ally going to progress to diabetes, what's the point in adding unnecessary stigma and stress—not to mention the expense of more frequent visits, tests, and possibly medications? Many public health organizations agree that an overly clinical approach to dia-betes prevention is ineffective. The WHO has argued instead for society-wide solutions aiming to address health impacts of social stratification, urban planning, and improved nutrition—all of which can affect the high sugar levels that are a trigger for the prediabetes diagnosis.

Root Causes of Diabetes

The feeling of shame in the room is palpable when I work one-on-one with clients who've been diagnosed with diabetes. There's often an urgency to "do better" and I'm frequently asked if the diagnosis can be reversed or the medication stopped with x and y change. There's a level of bargaining that comes from a feeling that they didn't do enough to stop the condition from impacting them—an attitude conditioned by the popular refrain that we need to take personal responsibility for our life outcomes. This refrain perpetuates that idea that we're to blame for our individual choices and habits if they're seen as "bad." Have you ever felt this way? I'm quick to reassure patients with these intrusive thoughts that there are many factors that impact the occurrence of diabetes, and choosing a salad over French fries may be the least of those factors.

Take a second to imagine a tree. To understand what factors are impacting the leaves of the tree, we have to look underground at the roots and the soil. To understand why diabetes impacts you or your family, we have to look at your roots as well. There are many known root causes of diabetes. Figure 2 provides you with a visual of the underlying innate and systemic factors that may have contributed to your risk of diabetes development. Do you recognize any of these factors as applicable to you?

- **Social determinants of health (SDOH):** This represents factors in our environment that influence our health, such as economic stability; education and health care access and quality; neighborhood and built environment; and social and community context (HHS n.d.). Higher educational attainment, income, occupational status, availability of full-service restaurants and grocery stores, social cohesion, and a living space that is more walkable and further away from highways are all factors associated with reduced diabetes risk. The converse is also true: low levels of education, income, job security, and housing stability along with higher levels of exposure to environmental contaminants, food insecurity, and racism are all correlated with poorer diabetes outcomes.

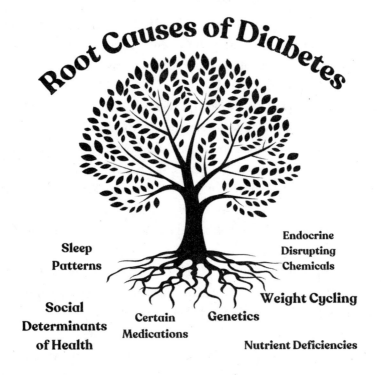

Figure 2

- **Disturbed sleep patterns:** The following are factors related to sleep that research has found are associated with diabetes risk:

    - Sleeping too much or too little. Seven to eight hours of sleep per day confers the lowest risk of diabetes (Shan et al. 2015).

- Night shift work (Pan et al. 2011; Vimalananda et al. 2015; Leproult et al. 2014; CDC 2015)

- Obstructive sleep apnea (OSA), which is a chronic sleep disorder that includes recurrent episodes of complete or partial obstruction of the upper airway, leading to intermittent hypoxemia (low levels of blood oxygen) and hypercapnia (high levels of carbon dioxide in the blood); brief and repetitive arousals from sleep; oxidative stress; and inflammation (Reutrakul and Mokhlesi 2017).

- **Use of certain medications:** Glucocorticoid drugs are used in nearly all medical subspecialties. While they offer benefits for certain medical conditions, there are also potential side effects, including steroid-induced diabetes mellitus (SIDM), which is an abnormal increase in blood glucose associated with using these meds when there was no prior history of diabetes. Factors that increase the risk for developing SIDM include the length of time on the drug, the potency, and the dosage (Hwang and Weiss 2014). Treatment of SIDM may require a different management strategy than non-SIDM, so talk to your health care team if you suspect your diabetes is SIDM.

- **Exposure to endocrine-disrupting chemicals (EDCs):** There is a body of evidence linking EDCs (BPA, phthalates/DEHP, PCBs, PFOA, DDT/DDE, TCDD) to an increased risk for T1DM, T2DM, and GDM in humans (Hinault et al. 2023). EDCs are aptly termed as they alter the production, release, transport, and action of hormones.

- **Genetic factors:** T2DM is associated with at least eight known biological mechanisms at this point in time (Defronzo 2009). In fact, there are a host of innate circumstances that influence diabetes development. Over the years, it has become increasingly clear that hyperglycemia resulting from T2DM is due to more factors than previously thought and there are actually many organs and systems involved. People destined to develop T2DM inherit a set of genes that make their tissues (liver and muscle) resistant to insulin.

- **Nutrient deficiencies:** A comprehensive 2020 review of studies using diverse populations from Asia, Africa, and North America validated the idea that micronutrient deficiencies may lead to oxidative stress and subsequently, insulin resistance and diabetes (Dubey, Thakur, and Chattopadhyay 2020). This topic will be discussed further in chapter 5.

- **Weight cycling:** When the pursuit of weight loss leads to restrictive eating habits (aka dieting), *weight cycling*—weight loss followed by subsequent weight gain—is a nearly guaranteed result. Weight cycling isn't to be taken lightly, as more and more studies are finding that body weight fluctuations lead to metabolic harm, including increasing diabetes risk. A 2021 review of fourteen studies with more than 250,000 people found that individuals who weight cycled had a 23 percent increased risk of developing diabetes (Zou et al. 2021).

We'll talk more about weight in the section that follows. First, take a second to reflect on all that you've just learned—ideally in writing, in your companion journal.

REFLECTION

- What type of diabetes do you have?

- Do you identify with any of the root causes of diabetes described? Has anyone ever mentioned these factors as potentially contributing to your diagnosis?

- Have you experienced judgment based on factors outside your control? How does this make you feel as a person with diabetes?

Diabetes and Weight

If you've been diagnosed with diabetes or prediabetes, I'd be willing to bet that at least one of your health care providers has insisted on weight management as the cornerstone to your treatment. Weight loss recommendations are handed out so freely at medical offices, you'd think a simple recipe for "success" existed. Yet, what we know about striving for intentional weight loss is that the overwhelming majority of people will only lose a small amount of weight in the short term before returning to their starting weight or higher. You read that right: data shows that nearly all dieters return to their starting weights within one to five years, and a majority of those dieters will actually be heavier in the end (Korkeila et al. 1999; NIH 1993; Stunkard and McClaren-Hume 1959). While there is absolutely nothing wrong with being in a larger body, it's pretty ironic that striving for a smaller body usually leads to the opposite of the intention. In addition, a number of studies have also demonstrated the ill effects of dieting and the nearly inevitable weight cycling that results. A large meta-analysis involving more than fourteen studies and over 250,000 subjects even found that weight cycling was a strong independent risk factor for new-onset diabetes (Zou et al. 2021)!

So why is weight loss such a commonly recommended treatment for blood glucose control? It seems to have all started with the body mass index (BMI) and the subsequent labeling of "obesity" as a disease. Let's explore this a bit.

The Birth of the "Obesity" Epidemic

The BMI's storied history begins in the 1800s with Belgian statistician Adolphe Quetelet. In 1832, Quetelet reported that body weight across adults varied with the square of height, which eventually became known as Quetelet's Index (Britannica 2024). He created this calculation to observe how weight was distributed across populations, but not to evaluate individuals and certainly not individual health.

At the turn of the 20th century, the American public began to focus more and more on body weight. Scales hit the market and people began purchasing them for home use, and doctor's offices began weighing patients at medical visits. In 1972, Ancel Keys, an up-and-coming researcher, published an influential paper making the case for a new body weight classification system. Keys found inspiration from Quetelet's Index and renamed it the body mass index (BMI) (Keys 1972). Because of his well-known work studying human starvation, diet, and heart disease, he was easily able to sway the American medical community to adopt the use of the BMI, despite the fact that the index was never intended to be used for individual health care. In the decades that followed, definitions and weight classifications continued to shape-shift, and potential conflicts of interest were rampant along the way. During this time, the National Institutes for Health (NIH) began by defining people as "overweight" or "obese" based on a weight percentile, not based on any particular health marker.

The next change to the weight standards occurred in 1998 when a panel of experts chosen by the NIH—many of whom had financial ties to the weight loss industry —voted to lower the BMI cutoffs, resulting in an additional 40 million Americans being given the title of "overweight" or "obese" overnight, despite having not gained a single pound. These changes were not in line with scientific evidence. In fact, the evidence supported *raising* the cutoff, as an association between BMI and mortality wasn't found until a BMI of higher than 40 (Brown 2015; Bacon 2010). The capitalistic gain from this change was clear as within two years, new weight-loss medications were approved and on the market with a wider reach of potential clientele. The new definition of who needed to lose weight offered the diet industry an expanded target market and larger customer base. Language surrounding the "obesity epidemic" and "war on obesity" also emerged, and the budgets for "obesity" programs at both the NIH and CDC increased significantly (Harrison 2019). In 2002, just one year after 9/11, Surgeon General Richard Carmona clearly aimed to strike fear in the American public when he described "obesity" as "the terror within, a threat that is every bit as real to America as the weapons of mass destruction." Unsurprisingly, he made the "obesity epidemic" a focal point in his work as Surgeon General.

In truth, Americans have gotten slightly heavier over the decades, but evidence to demonstrate that weight is causing disease or poor health is lacking. In fact, a study published in *JAMA* in 2005 found that moderately "overweight" individuals live longer than those at "normal" weights and that being "underweight" is much more dangerous (Flegal 2005). In his book *Fat Politics: The Real Story Behind America's Obesity Epidemic*, J. Eric Oliver states that "nearly all the warnings about 'obesity' are based on little more than loose statistical conjecture" (2006, 4).

Despite the lack of evidence to connect weight with cause for disease, in 2013, the American Medical Association (AMA) decided to label "obesity" as a disease, overriding a committee recommendation against this new classification (Pollack 2013). As a result, doctors were able to receive insurance reimbursement for "obesity" management, opening the door for a standard of *weight-normative care*—medical care that places undue focus on weight and weight loss as indicators of health and well-being (Tylka et al. 2014). With this new disease designation, doctors could now be paid to do things like prescribe weight loss drugs or perform irreversible surgery. Many in the medical and public health field soon found themselves benefiting from this new disease classification, including researchers who received funding to study new "obesity" drugs and doctors who were hired as highly paid consultants for weight loss companies.

The BMI categories also seem to distract some physicians from using clinical judgment, as evidenced by my client Cynthia. I began working with Cynthia while she was in remission from cancer and having a lot of side effects from surgery, chemo, and radiation. One such side effect was elevated blood sugar, which was in the range for diagnosis of diabetes. Yet her health care team was reluctant to diagnose her, instead urging her to lose weight and reverse course. Cynthia had frequently used steroids during her cancer treatment, a known risk factor for diabetes, yet her doctors focused on her weight because her BMI was outside the "normal range." I couldn't help but wonder if they would have the same treatment approach if she'd been in a smaller body, or if instead, they would have simply diagnosed her with diabetes per the ADA guidelines and prescribed a glucose-lowering medication. Instead, she experienced weight-biased care and delayed diabetes treatment, which harmed her health in a multitude of ways.

All size-based judgments are missing the mark—whether it's the BMI, the Body Roundness Index (BRI), a waist to hip ratio measurement, a visual appraisal, or something else. We cannot judge health by evaluating body size, body fat, or body weight as they are not health markers, nor are they behaviors. If you find your team is hung up on these metrics, we will discuss self-advocacy and partnering with your health care team in chapter 6.

Weight Loss Endeavors Cause Harm

A recent study published in *Diabetes Care* looked at the prevalence of diabetes among US adults from 2015 to 2020 and found that diabetes rates increased most significantly (17.8 percent) in adults with BMIs under 25 ("normal weight"), while there was only a 2.1 percent increase in the rate of diabetes in adults with "overweight" or "obese" BMIs during the time period (Adesoba and Brown 2023). Yet, as I'd bet you've experienced first-hand, when it comes to diabetes and weight, the common assumption and recommendation from health care providers is that weight loss aids diabetes control. Since most weight loss endeavors end in weight regain, this recommendation is both unhelpful and stigmatizing. In addition, the insulin resistance and metabolic changes that happen with T2DM—the type of diabetes most commonly associated with weight loss recommendations—make weight loss a near impossibility.

What happens if you try to lose weight with T2DM? A group of researchers from Denmark set out to study this. In the group of participants with T2DM who were "overweight" or "obese" by BMI standards, they found that weight loss, regardless of the intention, increased risk of death from all causes (Køster-Rasmussen et al. 2016)! In fact, the lowest rate of death was seen among those who *maintained* their weight during the nineteen-year study period.

In another large trial, which included sixteen centers in the US, the intention was to study the effects of calorie restriction and exercise on heart health in people with T2DM. The intervention group was to achieve and maintain a 7 percent weight loss by consuming a restrictive 1200 to 1800 calories daily plus doing 175 minutes of moderate-intensity physical activity per week. The study concluded that this intervention *didn't* reduce the risk of cardiovascular disease or death. In fact, the study was stopped early as the intervention was deemed futile (Look AHEAD Research Group 2013). Importantly, what was studied here is exactly what most health care providers have likely recommended you do—eat less and move more. Yet, this large-scale study demonstrated that following this overly simplistic advice likely won't yield the sought-after results.

Another recently published large study found that in healthy older adults, weight loss was associated with *increased* risk of disease, including an increased risk of cancer, cardiovascular disease, and other life-limiting conditions (Hussain et al. 2023).

Overall, these studies demonstrate that if you strive for intentional weight loss, you may be putting yourself at increased risk of death at worst, and a lack of weight loss "success" or improvement in any health outcomes at best. It doesn't seem like the potential benefit of attempted weight loss is anywhere close to outweighing (no pun intended!) the potential costs.

The Dangers of Weight Cycling

As you've read so far, evidence suggests that focusing on weight and striving for weight loss is harmful in a number of ways. In addition, we know that long-term weight loss isn't possible for most people (Bacon 2010; Tylka et al. 2014; Bacon and Aphramor 2011). What seems to be at the root of the poor outcomes and inability to sustain weight loss in dieters is *weight cycling.* Since diets don't actually "work" long-term, dieters tend to repeat their efforts to lose weight over and over again. Can you relate? If you've ever lost weight only for it to return and then doubled down on your efforts, you're not alone!

It's bad enough that weight loss is rarely sustainable, but even worse are the significant negative impacts on heart health and increased risk of death. In fact, weight cycling is nearly *guaranteed* to occur with each attempt at weight loss and is associated with negative medical, metabolic, and psychological health outcomes (O'Hara and Taylor 2018). Many research studies have demonstrated this point.

The ongoing Framingham Heart Study has studied over 5,000 people across three decades and found that weight cycling is significantly correlated with the occurrence of and death from coronary heart disease (Lissner et al. 1991). Similarly, a study out of Germany found an increased risk of death in *only* those whose weight fluctuated over the fifteen-year follow-up period. And, get this: the weight fluctuation was less than one BMI point! Just a few pounds can bump you one BMI point. For example, if you are five foot six, just a six-pound change will move you one point on the BMI chart. Of note, there was no increased risk of death found in participants with stable weights in the "obese" BMI range. In fact, those in the "obese" BMI group were not found to have higher risk than those in the "normal" BMI group (Rzehak et al. 2007). Another well-known, ongoing study called the Nurses' Health Study found that women with a history of weight cycling (39 percent of participants) were less physically active, had more binge-eating behaviors, and gained more weight compared with participants who didn't weight cycle (Field et al. 2004).

When it comes to diabetes and weight cycling, a number of studies have found harmful effects. One study looked at the health screening data of nearly 5,000 participants without diabetes and found that those with the most weight cycling over a four-year period were at significantly increased risk for diabetes development (Rhee et al. 2018). A Swedish study published in 2021 concluded that weight cycling predicts the development of cardiovascular complications in T2DM (Ceriello et al. 2021). Additionally, the results of a South Korean study, using nearly 4 million participants from Korea's National Health Insurance Service, suggest that weight cycling is an independent risk factor for diabetes. The researchers found this to be true even in participants under age 65 and who started the study with normal glucose tolerance status (Park et al. 2019). Yet another Korean study, published in 2020, concluded that weight cycling was associated with increased risk of heart attack, stroke, and all-cause mortality in patients with T2DM (Nam et al. 2020).

At this point, if you're scratching your head, wondering why we have such a weight-focused health care system when the evidence clearly doesn't support its use, you're not alone! Many of my clients over the years have asked me why their doctors continue to recommend weight loss despite its known futility, and even worse, its harms.

REFLECTION

- What treatments have you been through for diabetes?

- What messages have you received from doctors and others about weight loss, and how have they impacted your journey?

- Have you experienced weight cycling and its negative effects?

- What is your relationship with weight like? Your relationship with movement? How do you hope these might be healed?

If Not Weight, Then What?

You've likely been told your whole life that if you manage your weight, you'll be healthier, or if you lose weight, you'll improve your blood sugar and other health markers. You likely value health and want to feel healthy. Perhaps you picked up this book because striving for weight loss hasn't actually been as helpful as everyone claims it will be. Reading this chapter may have been shocking to you! You're likely wondering: if not weight, then what?

Maybe you're also wondering why doctors continually recommend weight loss in the name of "health" when there are clearly a host of ways that the pursuit of weight loss adversely affects health. Most health professionals have been trained to work within what's known as a weight-normative paradigm. *Weight-normative care*, which dominates Western health care practice, focuses on weight and weight loss as indicators of health and well-being. Conversely, *weight-inclusive care* emphasizes non-weight-based markers of health and well-being. Weight-inclusive care doesn't use body weight as the focal point of treatment or intervention (Tylka et al. 2014).

You're probably very familiar with the weight-normative care model. It's likely been used in every medical setting you've ever entered. In many outpatient medical practices, your weight is taken before you see the doctor regardless of whether your visit has anything to do with weight. (And truly, unless you are in need of a medication that is dosed based on weight or you have a condition in which dramatic weight changes indicate signs of a problem, such as congestive heart failure, there are few times that knowing one's body weight is actually necessary.) In our ultra-weight-focused health care system, you could be going in for a sore throat and still be asked to step on the scale!

Scholars have written about the consequences and shortcomings of the weight-normative model. The model has been described as contributing to anti-fat sentiment and weight stigma, increasing risks to health and well-being, worsening quality of life, and disregarding health promotion principles (O'Hara and Taylor 2018). In addition, the weight-normative approach may lead to food and body preoccupation, weight cycling, reduced self-esteem, or eating disorders, and is repeatedly unsuccessful at producing thinner or healthier individuals (Bacon and Aphramor 2011).

Weight-inclusive medical offices do exist, but unfortunately they are few and far between. Still, there are ways you can bring a more weight-inclusive approach to your diabetes care and your life. What I'll outline in the remaining chapters of this book are the ways in which you can care for yourself and your blood sugar without focusing on your weight. Health is never guaranteed, but there are many behaviors that we know can be health-enhancing. There are so many factors that may impact our health that have nothing to do with body weight: sleep, stress, nutrition, hydration, movement, human connection, environment, education, and socioeconomic status, to name a few. This is where we'll spend time, exploring the non-weight-focused ways that you can experiment with changes in your own life.

Moving Forward

Imagine letting go of the daily preoccupation with weight and dieting, and instead thinking about how you want to live and what would feel good for your body. Perhaps you can identify with the desire to want to manage blood sugar because it truly improves your energy, optimizes your sleep, and feels better in the day-to-day. Imagine improving your relationship with food, giving up the weight emphasis, and finding blood sugar benefits too. This is possible with a shift of focus, which is what intuitive eating for diabetes is all about. In the chapters that follow, I'll outline the four pillars of intuitive eating with diabetes and how you can create a diet-free lifestyle that isn't centered on what you weigh.

PART 1

The Four Pillars

CHAPTER 2

Pillar One: Establishing a Diet-Free Mindset

In this chapter, we'll be diving right into the first pillar of intuitive eating with diabetes: establishing a diet-free mindset. As you learned in the previous chapter, dieting and the pursuit of intentional weight loss often leads to harmful weight cycling. Contrary to mainstream messages, weight loss doesn't have to be part of how you manage your diabetes. Despite learning this, you may still struggle to accept that weight loss and food restriction aren't requirements for diabetes care. You may feel starkly anti-diet, yet still find the diet mentality creeping in sometimes. When the diet mentality has been the prominent way of relating to food—for any period of time—it becomes the ingrained way of thinking. Fortunately, our brains can be retrained to do things in new and improved ways, a concept known as *neuroplasticity*. Neuronal pathways are strengthened through repetition, so the more you engage with a diet-free mindset, the less often you'll be overcome by intrusive diet-mentality thoughts. It's hard work kicking diet culture to the curb, but it'll be worth the effort!

In this chapter, you'll be introduced to the ten principles of intuitive eating. You'll also have the opportunity to take the Intuitive Eating Scale (IES). The scale will highlight whether you are holding on to restrictive food practices, assess your level of emotion-based eating, uncover whether you trust your body's hunger and/or fullness signals, and determine how well you match your intake to what feels good for you. It'll give you a place to start in understanding intuitive eating and how it can work for you.

This chapter also includes an exploration of eating styles that undermine intuitive eating, and you'll have the chance to analyze whether your own patterns mirror any of the eating styles described. Finally, we discuss how the diet-free mindset supports us in intuitive eating for diabetes.

The Science on Intuitive Eating and Diabetes

The number of published research studies on intuitive eating has increased significantly since the concept was first written about in 1995. As of this writing, there are more than two hundred scientific publications on the topic. While there is a need for more focused research specifically looking at diabetes and intuitive eating, the studies that have been published to date have shown the promise that intuitive eating brings to diabetes management.

Several research studies have found the use of an intuitive eating framework to be a valuable tool for blood sugar improvement (Pires Soares et al. 2021; Wheeler et al. 2016; Willig et al. 2014). Tylka et al. (2019) found intuitive eating to be associated with greater weight stability, which is critical given the harms of weight cycling. Another study found that, regardless of BMI, intuitive eating was associated with an 89 percent lower chance of having poor glycemic control in people with T2DM that were not on insulin (Pires Soares et al. 2021). Yet another study found an association between intuitive eating and body satisfaction in patients with T2DM. Those who trusted hunger and satiety cues had body satisfaction levels twice as high as those that didn't trust those cues (Herzog Ramos et. al 2022).

In addition, other studies have shown that intuitive eaters have lower triglycerides and blood pressure, along with less body dissatisfaction and disordered eating. Intuitive eaters also have better HDL (good cholesterol) levels, higher self-esteem, greater food variety, enhanced life satisfaction, and more pleasure from eating (Tribole and Resch 2020).

In the past several years, Quansah and colleagues out of Switzerland have published three different studies looking at the effect of intuitive eating on GDM and diabetes postpartum. They've found that intuitive eaters had lower fasting glucose and HbA1c at one year postpartum, that intuitive eating may reduce the risk of developing diabetes postpartum, and a reliance on hunger and satiety cues was associated with increased insulin sensitivity (Quansah et al. 2019; Quansah et al. 2021; Quansah et al. 2022). In addition, an association was found between intuitive eating and increased diet quality and metabolic outcomes. All in all, really positive associations between intuitive eating and blood glucose control for women who had GDM in pregnancy!

Are You an Intuitive Eater?

The first Intuitive Eating Scale was developed in 2006, and since then has been through three iterations, with the newest revision published in 2024 (Tylka 2006; Tylka and Kroon Van Diest 2013; Tylka et al. 2024). The IES was developed and validated by researcher Tracy Tylka and her colleagues at Ohio State University as an initial tool to lead the research on intuitive eating, the ten-principle construct that Tribole and Resch first wrote about in 1995. As you'll see, it provides a personal assessment of four overarching intuitive eating domains. It's been adapted from its original format (Tylka et al. 2024) to a simple yes-or-no response for ease of use. Your results will highlight which areas of intuitive eating need some extra attention.

I invite you to go through the assessment with honesty and freedom from judgment. This scale aims to assess your approach to eating foods that are *available* to you—meaning foods you have access to, can afford, and don't have a medical or value-based reason for avoiding (such as a food allergy, religious or ethical reason, etc.). You'll be asked to answer yes or no to a variety of statements, and while you may be torn between the two options at times, simply aim to answer in line with what is true *most* of the time.

INTUITIVE EATING SCALE (IES)

Yes	No	Unconditional Permission to Eat
		I give myself the freedom to eat foods that I enjoy the taste of, without judgment.
		I allow myself to eat foods that taste good, without guilt.
		I eat foods that give me pleasure, without feeling ashamed about it.

Yes	No	Eating for Physical Reasons
		I eat when I am physically hungry more so than when I am feeling distressed.
		I generally eat to provide nourishment and fuel for my body more than to relieve emotional distress.
		My main ways of coping with distressing thoughts and feelings don't involve food.

Yes	No	Reliance on Internal Hunger and Satiety Cues
		I generally rely on my body's hunger signals to tell me when to eat.
		I generally rely on signals that my body is comfortably full to tell me when to stop eating.
		I pay attention to my body to tell me when, what, and how much to eat.

Yes	No	Body-Food Choice Congruence
		I prefer foods that give me lasting energy.
		I choose foods that help my body perform the best it can, both physically and mentally.
		I eat foods that feel good in my body.

Scoring

How many yes responses? _____

How many no responses? _____

What did you learn about your eating habits by taking the IES? The more yes responses you have, the more you are currently eating intuitively. If you responded no to some or all of the items, that's fine! Hopefully reading this book will help you address some of the ways in which you are not currently eating intuitively.

Tylka's research has demonstrated that intuitive eaters have an enhanced ability to perceive physical sensations that arise from within the body, which is known as *interoceptive awareness*. Intuitive eaters are able to both receive (interoceptive sensitivity) and act (interoceptive responsiveness) on internal cues from their bodies with regard to food. This may mean noticing and responding to hunger by seeking out food. It may be the ability to sense whether a food feels or tastes good. And while intuitive eaters may sometimes get overly full (we all do!), most of the time, their body awareness will lead them to eat until satisfied and pleasantly full.

If you're reading this and thinking that you aren't currently feeling connected to these sensations, that's okay! It may take some time to reconnect to your body. Removing obstacles to interoceptive awareness, such as the diet mentality, can start the shift in focus from external rules to internal sensations.

In a study examining the relationship between intuitive eating and glycemic control in adolescents with and without T1DM, it was found that those with T1DM had more emotion-based eating, which impacted their glycemic control (Wheeler et al. 2016). In addition, the adolescents with diabetes had lower intuitive eating scores on the IES than their peers without diabetes. These results are consistent with the findings of other researchers who studied individuals with T2DM. In general, these studies have found lower IES scores in people with both T1DM and T2DM. The diet mentality is likely at play in these individuals, thus impacting their level of unconditional permission to eat and their level of interoceptive awareness. The combination of a diet-free mindset and strengthening intuitive eating skills holds immense promise as a non-restrictive treatment option and a way to improve blood sugar.

Eating Styles

Tribole and Resch have described common eating personalities in their book, *Intuitive Eating: A Revolutionary Anti-Diet Approach* (2020). These eating styles include the careful clean eater, the professional dieter, the unconscious eater (with a few subtypes: chaotic unconscious eater, "refuse-not" unconscious eater, "waste-not" unconscious eater, emotional unconscious eater), and, finally, the intuitive eater. Check out the following examples and see if you can recognize any of the characteristics present in your own eating patterns.

The Careful Clean Eater

Description: Careful clean eaters are extremely particular about what they eat and have a perfectionistic interest in nutrition. They may exhibit signs of *orthorexia*, a disordered eating pattern that is characterized by an unhealthy obsession with healthy eating.

Case example: Marsha was scared into a rigid way of eating when she learned she had diabetes. Now, when she goes out to eat with her husband, she watches him enjoy a meal while she either brings along a low-carb yogurt or waits until she gets home to eat something she deems "safe" for her diabetes. Even though her lab results are now excellent, she is perpetually worried about how her food will impact her blood sugar.

The Professional Dieter

Description: The professional dieter is perpetually following the latest diet trend—and is often not shy about vocalizing it either. The goal of the dieter is to shrink their body in an attempt to meet the unrealistic thin-ideal standards of diet culture.

Case example: Marcus, age 45, has been on every diet imaginable and can tell you how many carbs, calories, or points are in any number of foods. He's in a constant battle with his body and is trying to manipulate his food intake to lose weight because he's been told that's the way to "reverse" his diabetes.* However, with each diet, Marcus becomes more preoccupied with food and his body, and he's actually trending up in weight. He's fed up with dieting, but he's just so confused about how to eat and worries about his health.

The Unconscious Eater

Description: The unconscious eater is akin to a distracted or mindless eater. This type of eater is often eating while doing another task, such as working at the computer or watching TV. The unconscious eater eats without awareness and may not actually realize how much or when they are eating. There are several subtypes of the unconscious eater.

Case example: Jenny, age thirty-one, works in a busy office environment. She often gets up to walk to a colleague's desk throughout the day and passes candy dishes that she snacks from along the way. In the break room, her co-workers often bring in donuts, bagels, and other items to share. Sometimes she finds herself nibbling on whatever's been left out without necessarily feeling hungry. At lunch time, she eats at her desk to multi-task and is surprised when she looks down to see that she's finished her meal without even realizing it, sometimes feeling stuffed after her food settles. Jenny's unconscious nibbling and lack of attention during meals negatively impacts her blood glucose. She gets really down on herself about her constant snacking and high blood sugar levels, but can't seem to figure out how to make a change.

---

* A note on "reversing" diabetes: Although there are various people and programs that promise this, research hasn't demonstrated this to be possible. Instead, diabetes can be controlled to within "normal" glucose values.

Subtypes:

The Chaotic Unconscious Eater

Description: A chaotic, disconnected eating pattern as a result of an overscheduled life. Eating is an afterthought and more of a reactionary, grab-and-go situation.

Case example: Monica, age thirty-six, a pharmaceutical sales rep and single mom of two, is always on the run driving from different medical offices throughout the county. The morning rush of getting her kids ready for school and making it to the first office by 9 a.m. often causes her to skip breakfast. By the time she drives through a neighborhood fast food restaurant for lunch, she's at a level of primal, extreme hunger. Monica often eats while driving and then feels overly full and uncomfortable. Between managing her home and work life, she feels completely overwhelmed and can't figure out how to take care of herself in addition to every-thing else.

The Refuse-Not Unconscious Eater

Description: This is someone who has trouble turning down food when offered despite a lack of hunger.

Case example: When Kenny was getting ready to visit family for the holidays, he shared with me that he was really dreading the Thanksgiving meal because he always feels pressured to try every-one's creations. He said, "In my family, food is love and it's consid-ered rude to turn it down, plus comforting home-cooked food tastes so good! I usually eat beyond my fullness cues and my blood sugar sees the effects of this."

The Waste-Not Unconscious Eater

Description: This type of eater is a member of the "clean plate club," meaning that they'll see a plate of food to completion without fully considering how they feel. Some parents who are apt to eat kids' leftovers as a means of not wasting the food despite a lack of hunger also fall into this category.

Case example: I met with Hillary after her doctor recommended nutrition counseling for her prediabetes. After our initial session, she spent some time trying to identify any unconscious food rules she had in place from years of dieting. At our next session, she said, "I noticed something very interesting about myself. I can't stand to waste food, but instead of simply saving a small amount of leftovers, I often just eat it right then and there. I have the thought that 'it's too much effort to find a container' or 'it'll just get lost in the fridge.' I treat my mouth like a trash can!"

The Emotional Unconscious Eater

Description: For this individual, stress, boredom, or feelings regularly impact eating.

Case example: Emerald reached out to me for help with her T2DM, which she had been managing on her own for four to five years. She also had a nearly twenty-year history with disordered eating, which began at age seven. She described a family health history that included an intergenerational legacy of eating disorders, diabetes, substance abuse, and mental illness. In addition to diabetes, Emerald was also diagnosed with generalized anxiety disorder. In our first meeting, she told me that she doesn't binge, but does use food to numb. She said, "Idle time is hard for me. I often find myself filling the space by eating."

The Intuitive Eater

Description: An intuitive eater makes food decisions that are in line with their internal cues. They have trust in their body's communication and a knowledge of their body's inner workings. This might mean eating when hungry, but could also mean eating based on knowledge of blood sugar patterns, as fuel before movement, or when there won't be another opportunity to eat for a while. An intuitive eater has learned which foods are satisfying for them and eats meals and snacks in a regular, nourishing pattern. However, an intuitive eater isn't a "perfect" eater, but rather one that aims to meet the body's needs and desires as best they can.

Case example: Daniel and I worked for a long time on breaking the diet mentality and bringing back innate intuitive eating skills that had been buried by decades of dieting. We even concluded our work together because he was doing so well. When he was diagnosed with SIDM about a year later, he requested to start meeting again because he was getting confusing food messages from his diabetes providers. In our second phase of work together, Daniel learned to apply the intuitive eating skills he already had to his new diabetes diagnosis. He honored his hunger and injected the appropriate amount of insulin for his intake. His blood glucose and HbA1c values drastically improved to within ADA goals in a matter of months. He continued to eat the foods he loved, in the amounts he desired, AND managed his diabetes by relying on his intuitive skills.

REFLECTION

- What type of eating style most closely resembles your own eating patterns? What has that been like for you?

- After taking the IES, what areas of intuitive eating stood out to you?

You Were Born an Intuitive Eater

Intuitive eating skills are innate for most people. If you've ever seen a typically developing infant eat, especially a breastfeeding infant, then you've seen intuitive eating in its purest, most original form. A nursing baby will signal hunger by putting fist to mouth, moving their head in search of a nipple, or crying (a late sign). If that baby is put to the mother's breast, they'll drink until their small but rapidly growing stomach is full, and then they'll stop. That's it. Neither baby nor mom will know how much was consumed, and it's nearly impossible to convince a baby with a full stomach to nurse more. This happens all over again in a few hours when the baby's hunger returns.

For many humans, the intuitive drive for food gets interrupted somewhere along the way. This may happen if a parent encourages a baby to drink a certain number of ounces out of a bottle or to consume a certain number of spoonfuls of pureed food. This interruption can occur when a child is told they need to take three more bites or that they must eat their veggies to earn dessert. Encouraging a certain volume, number of bites, or showing preference for a particular food (i.e., veggies over dessert) can cause intuitive eating skills to diminish. Instead of teaching a child to rely on their internal body wisdom, these interruptions tell them to look externally. These pressures to eat in line with parental expectations erode internal body trust.

Children are actually very good at eating to match their nutrition needs when undisturbed. Researcher Leann Birch and colleagues demonstrated this in a landmark study published in the *New England Journal of Medicine* in 1991. After measuring the twenty-four-hour energy intake of young children, ages two to five years, over six days, they concluded that the food consumption of children is highly variable from meal to meal but daily energy intake is relatively constant because the children *intuitively* adjust their intake as needed (Birch et al. 1991).

If you are an adult realizing that you've veered off your intuitive eating path, it's possible to get back on course. So many naturally born intuitive eaters drift off course because of family food rules, portion "control," weight regulation tactics, or other external controls on eating. A diagnosis of diabetes can introduce an additional layer of complication, leaving you to feel like your intake *must* be managed, and often by rigid rules, lest your blood sugar levels end up too high or too low. But the principles of intuitive eating are ones we can all learn to practice, at whatever age and under any number of conditions.

As mentioned, the ten principles of intuitive eating were originally defined by Tribole and Resch in their first edition of *Intuitive Eating* back in 1995. Below, I've outlined those principles with special consideration to diabetes management. An asterisk (*) marks those principles that aim to remove obstacles to interoceptive awareness . A double-asterisk (**) marks those principles that aim to improve interoceptive awareness.

- *Principle 1:* **Reject the Diet Mentality***

  The diet mentality is a mindset that over-values thinness and holds to a rigid view of what constitutes "healthy" eating for diabetes. Reject the diet mentality by saying no to food and body rules and yes to food flexibility and body peace. Diabetes treatment needs to be individualized and diets have no place here.

- *Principle 2:* **Honor Your Hunger****

  Keep your body nourished with regular, adequate meals and snacks. Help yourself achieve blood sugar stability by eating consistently throughout the day and honoring your hunger signals.

- *Principle 3:* **Make Peace with Food***

  Adopt an "all foods fit" mindset and let food preoccupations diminish. Contrary to common nutrition myths, there are no foods that are off limits for people with diabetes! Food restrictions create a feeling of scarcity, which often leads to unfavorable eating behaviors (such as out-of-control eating) when the food rule is temporarily bent.

- *Principle 4:* **Challenge the Diabetes Police***

  The diabetes police encourage binary, inflexible thinking about diabetes, food, nutrition, movement, self-monitoring, and medications. It categorizes actions within these topics as good and bad, healthy and unhealthy, right and wrong. To challenge the diabetes police, talk back! This may mean talking back to your own thoughts or to unhelpful comments and unsolicited advice from others.

- **Principle 5: Discover the Satisfaction Factor****

Have you ever eaten a meal or snack only to find yourself still searching for something to eat afterwards? It's possible that the eating experience or food was not satisfying. This commonly happens when people eat diabetes-targeted diet foods that aren't filling enough, don't taste great, or are eaten in a rush. Bring joy back to meals and snacks and aim to eat foods that have pleasing sensory properties to discover the satisfaction factor of intuitive eating.

- **Principle 6: Feel Your Fullness****

What does it feel like to be pleasantly full? It's okay if you're not sure. See if you can experiment with paying attention to different signs your body may give to signal that you're done: diminishing taste, slowing down, feeling less interest in your food, the physical feeling in your belly. Many people find it helpful to check in with the body partway through a meal to gauge how much more food they might want. (Note: Some diabetes medications and conditions impact the feeling of fullness. Discuss your specific situation with a trusted health care professional.)

- **Principle 7: Cope with Your Emotions with Kindness***

Sometimes food can feel like the perfect response to an emotion—be it boredom, sadness, or elation. Eating something comforting *can* be a kind way to treat the body when feeling down. However, it can't be the *only* way we know to treat our emotions. It's great to have a wide array of tools in our toolbox for helping us through our feelings, such as creating art, using sensory objects, or listening to a podcast or music. One important note to keep in mind: restrained eating that results in out-of-control eating is sometimes labeled as "emotional eating" when it's really just the result of primal hunger. (Hypoglycemia can lead to out-of-control eating as well.) If you've thought of yourself as someone who eats emotionally, can you get curious about whether you may have some restrained eating going on?

- *Principle 8:* **Respect Your Body***

  Imagine treating your here-and-now body with unconditional respect. Doesn't your body deserve to be taken care of, nourished, and treated with dignity? Some people experience anger toward their bodies for getting diabetes. It's understandable to feel frustrated or disappointed by this diagnosis. Can you accept the diagnosis without feeling that anyone or anything is at fault, and take good care of the body you have anyway?

- *Principle 9:* **Movement—Feel the Difference****

  There's no one way to move the body. You could move fast, slow, or in between. You could be sitting, standing, in the water, or on wheels. What's important here is that you find a way to move that feels good. Physical activity can be beneficial in just ten-minute spurts, and doing so is just as good as doing a longer duration all at once. Just ten minutes of any type of movement can reduce blood sugar spikes when done after meals (Buffey et al. 2022). Let's figure out what works best for you.

- *Principle 10:* **Honor Your Health with Gentle Nutrition***

  This principle captures a number of points: You can honor your health and eat the foods you love simultaneously. It takes eating a variety of food groups regularly throughout the day to nourish your body. There is no one right way to eat. People all over the globe use various cultural foods to nourish their bodies.

Developing a Diet-Free Mindset

If you've been on a diet at some point in your life, you're in the majority. What's dieting been like for you? I've never met someone who *likes* dieting. Most people I've worked with have restricted their food because they thought they had to in order to "be healthy." Now that you've learned that higher weights don't cause disease, that dieting leads to harmful weight cycling, that all foods can fit (even with a diabetes diagnosis), and that intuitive eating improves diabetes outcomes, are you ready to give up the dieting mindset for good? I hope you shouted a resounding "YES!" Let's get to it.

To develop a diet-free mindset, let's evaluate where diet culture is still influencing your thoughts or actions. *Diet culture* is a system of beliefs that glorifies thinness, criticizes certain ways of eating, encourages weight loss, and stigmatizes people who don't match societal or cultural expectations of what "health" supposedly looks like. Below are some ways many people engage with diet culture. Which are you currently doing?

- Avoiding certain foods or food groups in an attempt to eat fewer calories or to "be healthy"

- Stepping on the scale regularly

- Consuming media that promotes certain ways of eating: diet cookbooks, blogs, or magazines; social media—weight loss promoters, "wellness" influencers, or products

- Commenting on other people's bodies, saying things like "you look so good, have you lost weight?"

- Tracking food intake on an app

- Thinking of a meal or a day of eating as either good or bad, healthy or unhealthy

- A kitchen filled with "diet" foods

- Engaging in performative eating, where you eat differently around others than you would alone

- Privately or publicly criticizing your body or food choices

- Getting hung up on scrutinizing every inch of yourself in a photo

- Only showcasing older photos, where your body is different from your current body's size and shape

- Maintaining a closet full of old clothes *just in case* they fit again

If you've identified some ways that you're still in the diet mindset, perhaps you can begin moving toward a diet-free mindset with the help of a diet-culture overhaul:

- Throw out diet books, magazines, and recipes.

- Get rid of the scale.

- Clean out your closet—only keep what fits your body today. If you need new clothes, can you treat yourself to a few replacement items? Clothes shopping can be such a challenge for so many reasons—we'll discuss this further in chapter 8.

- Put pictures out that feature you in your body TODAY.

- Clean out your kitchen—get rid of diet foods.

- Evaluate your social media—unfollow diet and weight loss accounts or any account that doesn't make you feel good about yourself.

- Before opening a restaurant menu, ask yourself what you feel like eating; think about the temperature, taste, texture, mouthfeel, your hunger level. Then, open the menu and try ordering what you actually want to eat.

- When people around you engage in "diet talk," can you change the conversation topic or set a boundary by stating something like "I'm working on approaching food and body image differently now; can we talk about something else?"

This may be an intimidating list of changes to contemplate. It's okay to start with the steps that are easiest and work your way toward the steps that are harder; breaking free of diet culture is a process. See if making even one or two of the changes above helps you feel or act differently than you once did.

Case Example: Lily, the Professional Dieter

Lily started her professional dieting journey as a child. At the age of ten, she started attending Weight Watchers meetings with her mother. She watched her mom count food points all week long and attend weekly meetings to get weighed, where pounds lost would be celebrated and gains besmirched. She observed the willful struggle for thinness and the fight against fatness. As a larger-bodied child, she absorbed the message that her body was wrong and began dieting and counting points too. When I began working with her, she was in her forties and had been dieting for over three decades. In that time, her body had lost and gained weight dozens of times. Although she didn't want to continue counting points and going to meetings, she didn't know what else to do. She'd just been diagnosed with diabetes and her doctor prescribed metformin and weight loss. As a therapist, Lily was somewhat familiar with intuitive eating, but felt lost. Working to develop a diet-free mindset was the first step forward in our work together. Through critical analysis of her past dieting ways, she was able to determine that counting points and tracking her weight was only keeping her stuck, so she discontinued her Weight Watchers membership, got rid of too-small clothes, unfollowed weight loss Instagram influencers, got rid of her scale, and began experimenting with more enjoyable ways of nourishing herself. She was relieved to find that her blood sugar did well with these changes and she felt a sense of food freedom for the first time in her life.

Moving Forward

I hope you've been able to truly explore pillar one of intuitive eating for diabetes: establishing a diet-free mindset. Even if you've removed the tools of dieting from your life, you may still have thoughts that try to lead you back to your dieting ways. It takes time to truly disconnect and is especially challenging to do while living in a culture that normalizes and even celebrates dieting practices. Feel free to pause here while you work on disconnecting from diet culture. Perhaps you can use a calendar and schedule one action item each day or week from the listed ideas in the "diet-culture overhaul" in this chapter to help you move closer to a diet-free mindset. Spend some time connecting with how it feels (or will feel) to be free of diet culture's tools. When you're ready, move on to pillar two in the next chapter.

CHAPTER 3

Pillar Two: Diabetes Self-Care

Pillar two is all about self-care as it relates to diabetes management. *Self-care* is the process of attending to one's physiological and emotional needs, and is associated with enhanced physical health, emotional well-being, and mental health (Cook-Cottone 2015). Self-care isn't just about taking bubble baths and getting pedicures! It's an integral part of creating a lifestyle that includes health-promoting habits—and it has a real role to play in the care of diabetes. Building a sustainable self-care routine can also help you begin to get back in touch with your body when diet culture may have estranged you from it.

The Association of Diabetes Care & Education Specialists (ADCES) is a professional membership organization composed of nurses, dietitians, pharmacists, and other health professionals with the unified purpose of optimizing care for those with diabetes. ADCES has outlined seven self-care behaviors for people with diabetes, known as the ADCES7. These seven self-care behaviors include healthy coping, healthy eating, being active, taking medication, monitoring, reducing risk, and problem solving (Kolb 2021). Since ADCES isn't specifically aligned with intuitive eating or weight inclusivity, I have given these seven self-care behaviors an *Intuitive Eating for Diabetes* update below:

ADCES-7 Self-Care Behaviors
(adapted for use within the intuitive eating framework)

1. **Healthy coping:** Cope with the daily stresses of diabetes management through positive outlets, such as meditating, journaling, seeking support, or practicing a hobby that brings enjoyment.

2. **Healthy eating:** Practice intuitive eating by choosing a variety of nourishing foods in satisfying amounts.

3. **Being active:** Spend time moving your body in ways that bring joy. This can be structured or unstructured, and adapted for ability.

4. **Taking medication:** If you need medication, work with your health care team to determine which will be best for you. Be sure to ask questions about how to take the medication and what to do if you experience side effects.

5. **Monitoring:** Many people with diabetes are asked to monitor blood sugar and other metrics. Monitoring can provide useful information, but take care to notice any stress this practice brings on and discuss the level of monitoring that will work best for you with your team.

6. **Reducing risks:** Get screened for potential diabetes complications to reduce your risk factors. Screenings may include: regular medical checkups, eye exams, vaccinations, foot checks, mental health assessments, laboratory testing, dental care, sleep apnea screenings, and hearing tests.

7. **Problem solving:** Certain situations or outcomes may require some creative problem solving, such as a new work schedule, a vacation, or an illness. If possible, communicate with your health care team about the situation so that you can come up with a plan and test it out.

As you can see from the list above, diabetes management doesn't occur in a vacuum. It's not just about food or activity, as there are many factors that may affect blood sugar outcomes. As you read through the seven areas, did anything stand out to you as something you do well already, or that you'd like to improve upon?

Mindful Self-Care

Researcher Catherine Cook-Cottone has developed a mindful self-care scale aimed at addressing ten domains of self-care: nutrition/hydration, exercise, soothing strategies, self-awareness/mindfulness, rest, relationships, physical and medical practices, environmental factors, self-compassion, and spiritual practices (Cook-Cottone 2015). Here, I'll share with you some key questions to ponder about your own mindful self-care, influenced by Cook-Cottone's scale:

- Do you often take time to do something to **relax** (such as engaging in a creative activity like art, playing music, or listening to comforting sounds)?

- Do you frequently engage in activities that help you **physically care for your body** (such as eating a variety of nutritious foods, engaging in physical movement, or doing a mind/body practice)?

- Do you practice **self-compassion** by kindly acknowledging challenges and engaging in supportive self-talk?

- Are your **relationships** supportive? Do you feel respected, listened to, and encouraged?

- Are you **mindfully aware** of your thoughts, feelings, and body?

- Is there a **balance** between life's demands and things that are important to you?

Answering yes to the questions above is positively correlated with well-being, while negative responses are correlated with burnout. How many yeses did you have? How many nos? If you answered with mostly yeses, that's awesome—you are prioritizing self-care! If you answered with mostly nos, let's get curious about why that is and brainstorm some ways you may be able to flip some of those nos to yeses.

Let's take a closer look at some of the areas of self-care noted in the questions above.

Relaxation

There are a number of techniques that may help you relax, including diaphragmatic breathing and various mind-body practices.

Diaphragmatic Breathing

The diaphragm is a large muscle located at the base of your lungs and above your stomach. You can find it by putting three fingers above your belly button and taking a deep inhalation to feel your diaphragm move. Diaphragmatic breathing (also known as abdominal or belly breathing) is meant to help you use your diaphragm to take big, deep, effective breaths rather than shallow chest breathing. Diaphragmatic breathing allows the body to take in more oxygen and expel more carbon dioxide, which helps to lower both heart rate and blood pressure. In addition, breathing this way stimulates the vagus nerve and activates the relaxation response of the parasympathetic (rest and digest) nervous system. Over time, and with continued practice, additional benefits can be realized in core muscle stability, exercise tolerance, and injury reduction. Studies have found that when stress reduction and diaphragmatic breathing are added to conventional diabetes treatment, improvements are seen in both mental well-being and diabetes control (Yadav et al. 2021; Hegde et al. 2012; Fiskin and Sahin 2021).

Want to give it a try? (Note: if you have a lung condition, such as COPD or asthma, talk to your provider to see if this is a good option for you.) This breathing technique can be done sitting or lying down. You may want to try it while lying down to start before you progress to sitting. Practice a couple times per day if you can. This will strengthen your diaphragm muscles and will allow you more access to deeper and efficient breathing.

- *Step 1:* Lie on your back. You can prop a pillow under your knees if that's more comfortable.

- *Step 2:* Place one hand on your diaphragm, above your belly button, and the other on your chest.

- *Step 3:* Breathe in slowly through your nose. You should feel the hand over your diaphragm moving outward as it fills with air. The hand on your chest should remain still.

- *Step 4:* Through pursed lips, exhale slowly. You should notice the hand over your diaphragm moving in and the hand on your chest continuing to remain still (Cleveland Clinic 2022).

Mind-Body Practices

Mind-body practices include yoga, chiropractic and osteopathic manipulation, meditation, massage, acupuncture, tai chi, healing touch, hypnotherapy, and movement manipulation (McKennon 2000). Below is a brief synopsis of what is known about the use of some mind-body practices with diabetes:

- Meditation may be a useful adjunct for lifestyle modification and medication management of diabetes, and also may improve well-being (Priya and Kalra 2018). Meditation has been practiced for thousands of years and its benefits are well-known but underutilized in today's fast-paced culture. There are many types of meditation and many ways to get started if you want to give it a try. You could use an app or engage in a meditative practice through yoga or by simply taking an allotted number of minutes to focus on breathing and the present moment.

- Yoga may enhance glycemic control, improve lipids, and decrease blood pressure (Garrow and Egede 2006; Innes and Selfe 2016). If you are wondering how you're going to twist yourself into a pretzel, let me stop you there. Yoga is an ancient Hindu discipline that involves breath control, simple meditation, and movement through bodily postures. Western adaptations of the practice have taken it to various other extremes, but if you'd like to give it a try, you can check out a basic yoga class for beginners on YouTube or other sites, such as http://www.doyogawithme.com, where you can choose your level, style, and length of time. No uncomfortable pretzel shapes necessary!

- While acupuncture has been used to treat T2DM for two thousand years, there is still a lack of strong clinical evidence behind its use. One meta-analysis concluded that acupuncture could be recommended as a supplementary treatment, as it seems to contribute to reductions in fasting blood glucose, two-hour blood glucose, and HbA1c. However, the studies to date have been of small sample size and poor quality, and thus there is a need for larger, longer-term studies (Chen et al. 2019).

- Although there is limited clinical data on the topic, it is likely that music therapy and art therapy have a positive impact on diabetes outcomes (Witusik, Kaczmarek, and Pietras 2022; Mandel, Davis, and Secic 2013). Other conditions have seen positive effects from these therapies, and there is no perceived ill effect from their addition (Abushukur et al. 2022).

- Both progressive muscle relaxation (slowly tightening individual muscle groups in the body, then releasing the tension, all while noting bodily sensations) and mindfulness meditation had a positive impact on providing pain relief from diabetic peripheral neuropathic pain. Progressive muscle relaxation also appeared to have a beneficial effect on reducing fatigue (Izgu et al. 2020).

Physical Care

How well do you physically care for your body? Are you drinking enough water, eating food in adequate quantity and variety, and regularly engaging in enjoyable physical movement?

Fluids

Let's start with a discussion about water. Do you know how much water your body needs in a day? I often hear a lot of numbers thrown around, but the go-to reference for information about human nutrient needs is the dietary reference intakes (DRIs). According to the DRI, depending on sex or life stage, adults need between 2.7 liters (11 cups) and 3.8 liters (16 cups) of water per day (Otten, Hellwig, and Meyers 2006). This includes all water contained in food, beverages, and drinking water.

Foods highest in water content include fruits, vegetables, milk, and yogurt. It's estimated that about 20 percent of our fluid needs come from food, thus leaving us responsible for drinking the remaining nine to twelve cups as fluid. You may need more if you are in hot or humid weather, at altitude, exercising, losing fluid due to illness, or if you are pregnant or breastfeeding. Water, sparkling water, milk, and unsweetened tea or coffee count toward your fluid intake.

So, are you getting enough? If you're not sure, you could opt to keep track of your intake during a typical day. If you do find it challenging to meet your fluid needs, consider the following: what temperature do you prefer for beverages—ice cold, room temp, warm? Do you prefer to drink out of a cup, straw, spout, or mug? When you leave home, do you bring a portable bottle with you? When you're sitting in one place, do you have a beverage next to you? For myself, I've found that I definitely drink more water when it's ice cold and from a portable, insulated straw cup. What about you?

Food Intake

We will cover gentle nutrition—the practice of choosing food that both honors your health and taste preferences while also making you feel good—in the next chapter, but for now let's talk about food as a means of self-care. Are you offering yourself at least three meals per day that include a variety of foods that are nourishing and appealing to you? Feeding yourself is a means of caring for yourself. If you're currently struggling in this area, why is that? Perhaps you would benefit from planning out your meals and snacks, or from setting reminders, scheduling breaks, and giving yourself permission to stop what you're doing and eat. Just like a car can't run without fuel, neither can you! Fuel up—it's a means of self-care.

Here's how you can start: Within one hour of waking up, have your first meal. Then, let no more than four or five hours go by before having the next meal or snack, and so on. We'll talk more about specific foods and meal planning in chapter 4.

Movement

What's your relationship with movement like? You may be more familiar with the terms "exercise" or "physical activity," but I prefer the word "movement" because it broadly identifies a variety of ways to be active. I've worked with many clients over the years who have had various types of movement soured by negative past experiences. If that's the case for you, perhaps you'd benefit from a re-exploration of movement from a new perspective. Have you ever stopped to ask yourself what you actually like to do? For example, do you like to move outside or inside, with others or alone, first thing in the morning or later in the day?

Or perhaps you tell yourself if you don't have a certain amount of time to be active, then you might as well not do it. Keep in mind that ten minutes of movement, three times per day, has been found to be just as health-enhancing as thirty minutes all at once. Short bouts of movement are known as "exercise snacks." Francois et al. (2014) studied the effects of exercise snacks before meals on blood sugar in a small group of subjects and found it to be time-efficient and effective in improving glycemic control. Since then, many others have studied the effect of exercise snacks. Exercise snacks seem to be most effective on blood sugar when they interrupt prolonged bouts of sitting, are done right before or after meals, or use large muscle groups in activities such as walking, climbing stairs, or squats (Gao et al. 2024; Helleputte et al. 2023; Duvivier et al. 2017).

Diet culture may have skewed your perspective on movement, but it's possible to choose an activity that feels like self-care and not self-punishment. Take a look at the activity list that follows (a more comprehensive version of which is available for download at: https://www.IntuitiveEatingForDiabetes .com/resources). Are there any that sound interesting to you? Maybe you forgot all about some of the activities listed, or maybe you've never heard of others. Take a few minutes to explore with curiosity. If you have physical limitations, take note of the activities marked with a double asterisk** which may be nice options for certain limitations. Activities that require no special equipment, membership, or travel are marked with a single asterisk*.

- Arm ergometer**
- Barre classes
- Bowling
- Dancing*
- Dodgeball
- Flag football
- Gardening*
- Hiking
- Hula hooping
- Jumping rope
- Laser tag
- Kayaking
- Martial arts
- Mat Pilates*
- Ping Pong
- Playing with pets or kids*
- Rock climbing
- Swimming
- Trampoline
- Walking*
- Water aerobics**
- Weightlifting
- Yoga*,**
- Zumba*

My client Ruth, a busy forty-two-year-old attorney, found herself sitting much more than she liked. She'd tried to get back into exercise by getting a gym membership or planning to use her stationary bike at home, but she just never found the time. When we discussed the idea of joyful movement in a session together, something clicked for her. She realized she simply didn't find joy in biking to nowhere or being in a sweaty, cramped gym. When I threw out the idea of an adult soccer league—to bring her back to her youth, when she'd been a passionate soccer player—her face lit up. By the time we met the next week, she'd already joined a team and had her first practice. She was so excited to be moving her body in a way that brought her so much joy!

BEING ACTIVE WITH DIABETES

Physical activity has a myriad of benefits and is considered to be central to the management of diabetes. Being active helps meet therapeutic goals of diabetes management: optimal blood glucose, lipid and blood pressure levels, and prevention or delay of the development of chronic complications of diabetes (Balducci et al. 2014). It also helps build or maintain muscle, enhances mood, improves energy levels, keeps joints and muscles flexible, and more. Maintaining an active lifestyle contributes to improving quality of life for those with diabetes.

If you are thinking about starting a new type or amount of movement, you'll likely want to check in with your diabetes management team to be prepared. This is especially true if you have any diabetes complications, such as neuropathy, or if you use insulin. You'll want to know about any recommended modifications and a safety plan to prevent or treat hypoglycemia (see info box).

Physical activity causes your muscles to become more sensitive to glucose, so most people will see a decrease in blood sugar levels during or following activity. However, for some—especially those doing high-intensity activities, such as heavy weightlifting, sprinting, or competitive sports—blood sugar can increase following a workout. Stress hormones, such as adrenaline, are responsible for the blood sugar increases seen in

HYPOGLYCEMIA

Hypoglycemia is a blood sugar level under 70 mg/dL. The only way to know if you're experiencing low blood sugar is to test. If you use a continuous glucose monitor (CGM), you still want to confirm any reported lows from your device with a fingerstick. Symptoms of hypoglycemia include feeling shaky, anxious, sweaty; having the chills; becoming irritable or confused; experiencing a rapid heartbeat; feeling dizziness, hunger, or nausea; feeling sleepy or weak; or having a headache or blurred vision. If you experience these symptoms, it's best to test your blood sugar and then follow the 15-15 rule if it's under 70 mg/dL. The 15-15 rule goes like this:

1. **Take in 15 grams** of fast-acting carbohydrate, such as any one of the following: 4 oz juice, 4 oz regular soda, 1 glucose gel, 4 glucose tabs, or 1 Tbsp of sugar or honey. (Don't use mixed foods containing protein, fat or fiber here—they take longer to digest and thus will be a slower means of raising blood sugar. Unless there's no other option, refrain from foods like candy bars and ice cream when you need to get your blood sugar up in a hurry!)

2. **Wait 15 minutes** and then re-test. If blood sugar is still under 70, repeat with another 15 grams of fast-acting carbohydrates. If it's over 70, proceed with the meal or snack you're due for.

Hypoglycemia happens more often in individuals using insulin or insulin secretagogues. In addition, hypoglycemia may occur in those changing their activity level, as the glucose-lowering effects of exercise can last up to forty-eight hours following the activity. For this reason, if possible, monitor a bit more frequently until you better understand how different types and amounts of activity affect your own blood sugar.

those engaging in more intense activity. This is all manageable once you learn your own personal responses to physical activity.

In general, it's best to make sure you've had a meal or snack at least 1 to 2 hours before activity if you plan to be active for more than 15 to 20 minutes. If you plan to be active for longer than 45 minutes, I'd recommend bringing a snack along with you. After 45 to 60 minutes of endurance activity, most people are running out of their body's stored fuel (glycogen), which can make hypoglycemia more likely. Again, we'll talk more about nutrition in the next chapter.

Self-Compassion

Self-compassion can be described as treating yourself with the kindness and understanding you would show to your own loved ones, especially during times of hardship. Several studies have shown that practicing self-compassion may improve the management of chronic conditions, including diabetes (Ferrari, Dal Cin, and Steele 2017). In a review of sixteen studies across the globe, self-compassion was associated with improved diabetes outcomes. In addition, it was found that self-compassion could be improved upon through intervention, meaning patients who didn't feel very self-compassionate at the start of the study felt more so by the end. Higher levels of self-compassion also led to more effective self-management behaviors, better glucose control, more optimal HbA1c levels, and greater life satisfaction (Sandham and Deacon 2023).

Self-compassion can act as an important psychological cushion in the face of diabetes-related mishaps, such as forgetting a medication or blood sugar being out of ideal range. A self-compassionate response to a mishap would embrace flexible thinking and offer understanding, such as "others also struggle with this," or "I'm disappointed that this happened, *and* I can forgive myself and do better next time" (Tanenbaum et al. 2018).

I invite you to take a moment to recall a recent diabetes mishap or disappointment you experienced. How did you talk to yourself? Was your internal communication kind? Overall, how self-compassionate are you?

The following examples demonstrate what it might look like to have self-compassion in the context of diabetes.

- I try to be gentle toward myself when I'm feeling down about my diabetes.

- When I'm going through a hard time with my diabetes, I give myself extra care and tenderness.

- I'm tolerant of my own flaws in managing my diabetes.

- I recognize that everyone struggles from time to time.

Supportive Relationships

Social support can be formal, coming from professionals and organizations, and informal, from loved ones, peers, or family members. It is the perception of being cared for and accepted. A number of studies have evaluated the relationship between social support and the impact on diabetes. Social support is correlated with improved diabetes clinical outcomes (HbA1c, blood pressure, lipids), improved diagnosis acceptance, enhanced blood sugar control, greater treatment adherence, decreased stress, and better quality of life (Strom and Egede 2012).

What is the level of social support like in your life? What has your experience with support and diabetes outcomes been like? Maybe you'd like to experiment with some new forms of social support but don't know where to start. If so, I've listed some ideas for formal and informal support below.

Formal: outpatient clinic diabetes group, telephone support, religious community group, senior center, neighborhood diabetes walk or event, group therapy

Informal: family, friends, peers, teachers, coaches, clergy

Mindful Awareness

If you face significant negative emotions related to your diagnosis of diabetes, you might be experiencing what's known as diabetes-related distress (DRD). DRD may include: fear of complications or adverse health outcomes, feeling overwhelmed from self-management demands, frustration from unresponsive providers, feeling angry or discouraged, isolation from unsupportive relationships, and/or worries about your ability to maintain a "healthy" lifestyle (Gonzalez, Fisher, and Polonsky 2011). Research studies have found DRD to negatively affect medication-taking, physical activity, food intake, and HbA1c levels (Bogusch and O'Brien 2019). However, mindfulness may improve quality of life and reduce DRD. *Mindfulness* is a practice of present-moment awareness, without interpretation or judgment. Learning how to practice mindfulness may involve breathing techniques, meditation, guided imagery, journaling, or other mind-body connection practices. Mindfulness interventions have shown promise in relation to a broad range of diabetes outcomes. If you're interested in adding a mindfulness practice to your life, here are some to consider:

- Use a guided meditation app such as Healthy Minds Program (free!), Calm, Insight Timer, Headspace, or Ten Percent Happier.

- Regularly practice journaling, doodling, or coloring.

- Spend time in nature. While there, connect with your senses. What do you see, hear, smell, feel?

- Disconnect from tech. Turn off your notifications and allow yourself to spend some time free from interruption.

- Use an inspiring meditative mantra with repetitive sounds or sayings to help the mind refocus. Here's an example: *My body is working hard for me each and every day. I'm grateful for what my body can do for me.* See if you can come up with a message of gratitude that feels true to you.

- Include a mindful minute for reflection before starting a meal. Look at your plate. Take in the colors and aromas. Consider your food's origin and the effort it took to get it to the state of preparation it's in as it sits on your plate. Give thanks to all of the people who contributed to your meal: the farmers, laborers, truck drivers, grocery workers, and cooks that helped your food get to you. Before you start to eat, connect with your hunger level. As you take your first bite, take time to chew and explore the sensory characteristics of the bite. As you continue to eat, check in with your hunger and fullness sensations. What do you notice? How will you know when you've had enough?

Balance

Does it feel like there are an insurmountable number of things to do to keep your diabetes in check and play an active role in family and work life? I feel you. To attempt to find some balance between life's demands and things that are important to you, I invite you to do a values assessment exercise (Stoddard and Afari 2014). Here's how it works.

1. Visit: https://www.IntuitiveEatingForDiabetes.com/resources to download the full values list. I've included an abbreviated list below. The goal is to identify a few of your top values: characteristics like "adventure," "compassion," "freedom," "strength," and more, that you might seek to practice or bring to your life.

2. Look over the list and identify no more than four that click with you. You may want to first start with a larger list and then narrow it down from there.

3. Then, write those top four selected values down in your companion journal. After you've done that, look at your first

identified value and ask yourself: on a scale of 1 to 5, how aligned am I with this value that I've identified as important to me (5 being most aligned, 1 being least aligned)?

4. From there, answer the following: What is contributing to this level of alignment? Is there anything I'd like to change?

5. Repeat this questioning with each of your identified values.

Values List

Compassion	Intuition	Self-sufficiency
Courage	Patience	
Creativity	Peace	Simplicity
Excitement	Perseverance	Spirituality
Fun	Reliability	Spontaneity
Health	Respect	Strength
Humor	Self-expression	Structure
Integrity		Wisdom

This values assessment exercise comes from acceptance and commitment therapy (ACT), a behavioral therapy that centers on valued engagement in life. I often use this exercise with clients who are feeling stuck in some way. Many find it helpful to connect with their values to reveal actions they're taking that are out of alignment with personal values and more in line with diet culture. For example, my client Rosie found that connectedness was very important to her, but her action of saying no to social outings involving food was leaving her feeling disconnected. Once she discovered the mismatch, we were able to work through what she'd need to live in a way that was more aligned with her value of connectedness.

REFLECTION

We've covered quite a bit in this chapter, outlining several areas of self-care to consider and a variety of strategies you can practice in each. See below for a rundown.

- **Relaxation:** diaphragmatic breathing; mind-body practices

- **Physical care:** adequate fluid; regular and balanced food intake; consistent and joyful practice of movement; blood sugar awareness

- **Self-compassion:** thinking in self-compassionate rather than self-critical ways, especially when you go through mishaps or challenges with your diabetes care

- **Supportive relationships:** pursuing relationships, whether in formal settings or in day-to-day life, that nourish you and don't reinforce diet culture's punitive, weight-normative messaging

- **Balance:** regular practice of mindfulness or other strategies to manage diabetes-related distress and the pursuit of actions that speak to what you truly value

Can you identify a particular area of self-care you'd like to improve? What are one to two things you can implement with at least 80 percent confidence to improve this area of self-care? If you'd like to track what you try and the results of the practice, you can do so with the tracking worksheet available at: https://www.IntuitiveEating ForDiabetes.com/resources.

Moving Forward

In this chapter, you've been able to explore pillar two of intuitive eating for diabetes: compassionate self-care. I hope you've been able to identify the many unique and varied ways you can care for yourself and your diabetes. You certainly don't have to do everything discussed in this chapter, but perhaps you can choose a couple things to either continue doing or to add on that will enhance your well-being. Look to be diverse in your self-care actions. Spend some time engaging with the compassionate self-care practices you've identified as important to you before moving on to the next chapter, pillar three—gentle nutrition.

CHAPTER 4

Pillar Three: Gentle Nutrition

In this chapter, I'll review the third pillar of intuitive eating for diabetes care, gentle nutrition. "Honor your health with gentle nutrition" is also the tenth principle of intuitive eating. It's the final principle, and for good reason. Without establishing a diet-free mindset and identifying ways to care for yourself in line with your values, you're likely to take in information about nutrition in a much different way. And if a positive relationship with food isn't in place, then eating for optimal nourishment becomes nearly impossible.

Now that you've begun the work of establishing a diet-free mindset, and you've evaluated the multitude of ways to take care of your body, we can dive into gentle nutrition. Gentle nutrition is about choosing food that honors your health and taste preferences while also making you feel good. It's not about weight loss or following food rules. In this chapter, you'll learn how to use intuitive eating skills and nutrition science to guide you toward satisfying, nourishing food choices, even as you continue to care for yourself and manage your diabetes. In addition, this chapter will include a detailed discussion of balanced meal planning; how interoceptive awareness informs hunger, satisfaction, and fullness; nonnutritive sweeteners; the glycemic index and load; carbohydrate-containing foods; cultural foods; and the nutrition facts label. Our discussion of gentle nutrition will include the use of five intuitive eating for diabetes principles: honor your hunger, make peace with food, challenge the diabetes police, discover the satisfaction factor, and feel your fullness.

Are You Hungry?

What signs does your body give you when you need food? In chapter 2, you were introduced to the bodily phenomenon known as interoceptive awareness, the ability to perceive physical sensations that arise from the body. Our bodies are constantly communicating with us in various ways. For example, when your bladder is full, your brain interprets this as the need to use the restroom. When your eyelids start to feel heavy, you know that you're sleepy.

When you feel hunger, your body will also communicate the need to eat with you. While a full bladder or sleepiness may have very obvious and specific signs, hunger may be perceived in a number of ways. The following are the variety of ways that people often experience hunger:

- rumbling stomach

- headache

- thirst

- lack of energy

- moodiness (aka being "hangry")

- thinking about food

- shakiness

- low blood sugar

What signs do you experience? If you're not sure, that's okay. If you've ignored your cues in the past, your distinctive hunger cues may be temporarily silenced. Hunger silencing may result for a number of reasons, including past dieting, stress, a chaotic schedule leading to skipped meals, or tricking your body's hunger pangs with calorie-free beverages, chewing gum, or "air foods" (such as rice cakes) that offer volume but not satisfying nourishment.

You can start to honor your hunger by looking for signs that you are hungry. You can use the hunger/fullness scale below to see if you can identify the described sensations in your own body. Regardless of how well you sense hunger now, you'll likely improve your awareness by ensuring you're eating regularly and avoiding some of the culprits of hunger silencing.

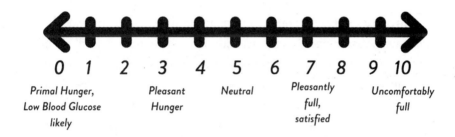

| 0 | 1 | 2 | 3 | 4 | 5 | 6 | 7 | 8 | 9 | 10 |

Primal Hunger, Low Blood Glucose likely — Pleasant Hunger — Neutral — Pleasantly full, satisfied — Uncomfortably full

On the scale above, the most intense level of hunger is a zero out of ten. This level of hunger is extreme, unpleasant primal hunger. With or without diabetes, primal hunger is often accompanied by low blood glucose (hypoglycemia). Many people will describe this hunger as urgent and desperate. For Mario, a client I worked with, when he felt the symptoms of primal hunger come on, his actions took place without thinking (brain fog or confusion is a symptom of hypoglycemia). In his fed state, he knew all about the 15-15 rule, but in his starved state, he'd grab candy and eat until the discomfort went away. That meant he'd often overdo it to the point of feeling overly full (level ten out of ten on the scale) and a rebound high blood glucose (hyperglycemia) would result. To prevent getting overly hungry, Mario learned that he needed to eat a variety of foods from all food groups regularly, allowing no more than four to five hours to pass between a meal or snack.

I've had many clients with dieting histories tell me they never feel hungry or they don't notice hunger until it's extreme. This is far too common when there's a history of food restriction. Many times, this feeling of primal hunger leads to a strong desire to eat carbohydrate-rich food. This makes sense since under-eating leads to the release of an appetite-stimulating chemical in the brain called neuropeptide Y (NPY). NPY causes the body to seek out carb-rich foods. NPY levels ramp up after any chunk of time without food, so levels are naturally highest in the morning, after your overnight fast. Because of this, skipping the morning meal can backfire and lead to primal hunger and subsequent rebound eating. The drive for carbohydrates is a protective one; since the brain feeds on glucose, carbs are the preferred means of receiving energy.

To avoid hunger extremes, most people feel best by eating a meal when their subjective hunger level is around three out of ten—a level we might describe as *pleasant hunger*. It may take some time to determine what pleasant hunger feels like to you. In general, think of this as a hunger that still allows you to calmly and patiently sit down to a mindful meal, rather than a rushed, urgent hunger. This may require a bit of planning ahead and getting to know your typical patterns. For example, Brooke found that because of her work schedule, she needed to eat before she was truly hungry to avoid getting overly ravenous. As a university dean, she often had meetings scheduled back-to-back for many hours on end. During her meeting marathons, she barely had enough time to use the restroom, let alone eat a meal. As a result, she decided to experiment with the idea of *practical hunger*. Since her meetings usually went from 11 a.m. to 4 p.m., she began eating lunch at 10:30 a.m. so that she could enter her long stretch of meetings well fueled. She also wisely kept a yogurt smoothie in her office fridge so she could have a sustaining snack a few hours later that wouldn't make a lot of noise or distract from her Zoom meetings. This strategy allowed Brooke to keep her energy and blood sugar levels stable during her long days of meetings.

This approach also works well for anyone taking a medication that blunts appetite or for those who are not quite in touch with their hunger cues yet (such as someone in recovery from an eating disorder). I often provide the following analogy to my clients: If you were going on a four-hundred-mile road trip, and your car's gas tank could take you three hundred miles but the fuel level was still indicating full at nearly three hundred miles traveled, would you keep driving or would you assume your gas gauge was broken and stop to fill up the car anyway? This can be applied to our food intake as well. If you've gone more than four or five hours without food and are still not noticing signs of hunger, can you be curious about why that might be? Many people benefit from setting phone alerts to remind them to eat, which helps to avoid hypoglycemia and/or extreme hunger later when hunger comes back online.

What Are You Hungry For?

Once you've determined that you're hungry or that it's time to eat, how do you decide *what* you want to eat? Satisfaction is the central tenet of intuitive eating, from which all other principles follow. When you consider satisfaction, you give thought to what will taste good in addition to what will sustain you. Consider the following sensory properties:

- Do you want something that **tastes** savory, sweet, salty, buttery, rich, sour, tart, smoky, spicy, bland, or mild?

- Do you desire a particular **texture**—smooth, creamy, crunchy, chewy, crispy, soft, flakey, gooey, mushy, sticky, or dry?

- Is there an **aroma** you are looking for?

- What food **temperature** is most appealing at this moment? Warm, room temp, cold?

- What **appearance** is calling to you? A vibrantly colorful plate or something uncomplicated and plain?

- How much **filling capacity** do you need this meal or snack to provide?

If you've never put this much thought into your meals, this may feel like an overwhelming amount of attention to pay to your food choices. As a more seasoned intuitive eater, these considerations will simply happen naturally, without much extra thinking involved. To practice, try this: the next time you're ordering food from a restaurant, stop to ask yourself what sensory characteristics you desire before you even look at the menu. For example, if it's a cold rainy day, maybe you want something warm and comforting, like a bowl of savory soup and buttery bread. Or if it's blazing hot outside, maybe you're in the mood for a cold sandwich, poke bowl, or salad. The key is to order based on your own desires and not to compare your food order to anyone else's. You are the only one who knows what your body truly wants and needs.

In addition to the sensory properties, can you think about what environment you find most pleasant to eat in? My client Julia always ate at her desk during her lunchtime at work. The problem was that she was constantly interrupted: colleagues would come into her office, her phone would ring, she'd get distracted by a seemingly urgent email. She wasn't truly giving herself a break and she was not able to mindfully attend to her meal. When we brainstormed the idea of relocating during her lunch break, she remembered that her office building has a nice outside area with tables and chairs. When she began taking her lunch outside, she realized how much nicer it was to get some fresh air and sunshine. She was thrilled because she was able to actually eat her meal with intention and she got a mood boost from her time outside. She found that eating with awareness greatly enhanced her meal satisfaction and actually led to a more efficient workday.

What does it mean to enjoy your food? How do you want to feel at the end of a meal? The chaotic unconscious eating style described in chapter 2 is a way of eating that has manifested due to the fast-paced way of life in many parts of the world. If you find yourself dissatisfied at the end of a meal, I invite you to try the practice below at your next meal. You likely won't be able to do this practice at every meal, but engaging with these steps a few times per week (or however often you find reasonable) can help you to foster more meal satisfaction.

1. After you've decided that you are pleasantly hungry and you know what you'd like to eat based on the desired sensory characteristics above, plate your food in an aesthetically

pleasing manner and choose a calm, comfortable, distraction-free place to sit down and eat.

2. Before you begin, take a few slow, diaphragmatic breaths to calm your nervous system. You may close your eyes, or simply find a non-moving spot to focus your gaze. Aim to cultivate gratitude for the meal before you start. Consider the steps your food went through to take the form of the meal before you: where and how it was grown, who labored to harvest ingredients, how it arrived in your kitchen and onto your plate.

3. Consider some additional ways to enhance meal satisfaction: keep conflict away from the table; include a variety of colors on your plate; and, if possible, don't settle: if you love it, eat it; if you don't, leave it.

4. Deeply inhale to take in the aroma of your food. How does it smell?

5. Get ready to eat. Prepare a small bite of food, and as it enters your mouth, let it move around a bit before you chew and swallow. How is the taste?

6. Continue eating in a manner that feels comfortable and pleasant to you.

7. Check in partway through the meal. Has anything changed about the taste of the food? *Sensory-specific satiety* is the point at which the desire or subjective liking of a food decreases during the course of eating it. Are you noticing any signs of fullness? Do you need to pause for a moment to let things settle before deciding if you'd like to continue?

8. If you're still hungry and it still tastes good to you, continue eating until you are pleasantly full (about a seven out of ten on the hunger/fullness scale, or when you notice diminishing

taste, slowing down, feeling less interest in your food, or a gentle fullness in your belly).

Once you try the steps above, I invite you to reflect on what you noticed. How was eating in this connected, mindful manner different or similar to the way in which you would typically have a meal? Maybe it was painstaking to pay that much attention to all those details! Are there any components of this practice that you'd like to keep in your mealtime routine? If so, consider how you'd like to incorporate them during future meals. You can make this process your own—that's what intuitive eating is all about.

Make Peace with Food

I've had countless interactions with people who have said, "I can't eat that. I have diabetes." When I hear this, I often wonder if the person saying it really means "I'm scared to eat this" or "I've made a rule to not eat this," because unless an allergy exists, there's really no food that someone with diabetes *can't* eat. I've had many clients also tell me that they don't keep certain foods in the house because they don't trust themselves around the food item. Do you have any foods that you avoid? What happens when that food is suddenly around?

If I were a betting person, I'd venture to guess that if you've had food rules or restrictions, then you've also experienced something known as *rebound eating*. If you imagine that restriction of a food is akin to a rubber band being stretched to its capacity, rebound eating is what happens when you let go of the rubber band—an unavoidable, forceful release occurs. Researchers Polivy and Herman (1980) referred to this as the *what-the-hell effect*. They saw that when a food rule was broken, the common response was to throw in the towel, as in *What the hell, I've already given in, so I might as well just keep going*. This is the inherent problem with food rules—they contribute to *all-or-nothing* thinking. Here are some examples of all-or-nothing thinking I often hear:

- I either eat "healthy" or "unhealthy."

- I'm either checking my blood glucose regularly or I'll go weeks without checking.

- I'm either going to the gym every day religiously or skipping all exercise for weeks at a time.

- If I'm not dieting, then I'm eating whatever I want without regard.

Do you sometimes have thoughts like these? All-or-nothing thinking is a cognitive distortion that involves thinking in extremes or absolutes. *Cognitive restructuring* is a process by which you can try to find some gray area rather than just the black-and-white, binary way of viewing a situation. For example, if we take each of the binary statements above and reframe them, here's what we might get instead:

- I can aim to eat a variety of nourishing foods *and* some fun foods with my meals, e.g. a sandwich with sides of fruit and chips.

- I forgot to check my blood glucose this morning, but I can check it before the next time I eat.

- I'm not able to make it to my favorite dance class today, so I'll go on a walk during my lunch break instead.

- I can allow myself to eat all foods in a way that feels good.

Deprivation leads to rebound eating. In addition, just the perception of an upcoming food restriction can lead to *last supper mentality*. This often happens before a new client comes in to see me. Even if I've spoken to them on the phone and told them that I use an all-foods-fit philosophy, inevitably new clients will eat the foods they fear will be taken away in excess amounts the night before our meeting. They view this as the last hurrah before they have to change their ways. In reality, when you give yourself unconditional permission to eat the type and amount of food that feels good, habituation is a likely result. *Habituation theory* proposes that repeated exposure to a specific food leads to a diminished response to the sensory properties of the food and thus less interest in that particular food (Swithers and Hall 1994; Ernst and Epstein 2002; Epstein et al. 2009).

Habituation happens when you become used to a food after regular, consistent intake of it. A food you've habituated to is no longer a big deal because you know you can have it anytime. Children's actions around food often provide great examples of this. If you've ever been to a kid's birthday party, you've likely observed which kids were food preoccupied and which were not. The children who don't have regular access to party foods may eat a lot of those foods at a party because they don't know when they'll have the opportunity again. Those who couldn't care less about the chips and birthday cake likely have regular access to those foods—they are habituated to them.

The more you allow yourself regular judgment-free but attuned access to your favorite foods, the more you'll habituate to them as well. But watch out for pseudo-permission, which is when you're eating the food but *telling yourself* that what you're eating is bad or wrong. Here's how you might start working on decreasing the allure of certain foods by allowing more permission:

1. Make a list of foods you either don't allow yourself to eat, feel bad about eating, or think you shouldn't eat.

2. Decide on one of those foods to bring into your home.

3. Include this food in your regular, consistent meals as often as you'd like. Give yourself permission to eat this food in a way that feels good to you. Depending on what the food is, you might include it daily or a couple times each week.

4. Repeat until you feel neutral to the food and think you can honestly honor your desire for it with full permission.

When my client Greg worked through this exercise, he decided to start with Chinese takeout. Typically, when ordering this food, he'd order all of his favorites and eat until he was overly full. He'd then enter a shame spiral. He'd tell himself he was bad for eating this food, that it was

CAN YOU BE ADDICTED TO FOOD?

I've had many clients tell me that they are addicted to food. I absolutely believe that these clients *feel* addicted to food, but I'm fairly certain that they aren't in fact addicted. We need food to survive, unlike those with alcohol or drug addiction who actually *need* to abstain from alcohol and drugs to survive. Here's what we know about this topic so far.

Food addiction research relies on the Yale Food Addiction Scale, which is a questionnaire that fails to take food restriction from dieting, an eating disorder, or low accessibility into account. Some have proposed that perhaps the scale is measuring dieting difficulties and binge eating rather than true addiction.

Animal research that supposedly demonstrates the addictive power of sugar was done on rodents who consumed sugar in an "addictive-like" way only when they were given intermittent access to it. Those rodents with unlimited access to the sugar didn't behave in this way. Intermittent access is the same as dieting or other forms of food restriction. When people are given unpredictable access to food, they behave in an "addictive" way too, but when they are given unconditional permission to eat, they don't.

Some claims that food is addictive argue that the same brain regions light up with highly palatable foods just like they do for drugs. However, there are many activities that can cause these reward centers in the brain to light up, such as puppies, babies, and music.

In 2016, a group of researchers published "Sugar Addiction: The State of the Science" and concluded that "there is little evidence to support [the idea of] sugar addiction in humans" and that the addiction-like behaviors occur only due to intermittent access to sweet, highly palatable foods, not the neurochemical effects of sugar (Westwater, Fletcher, and Ziauddeen 2016, 55). This research supports intuitive eating principles that aim to remove restriction and ultimately make peace with food.

unhealthy, and since he clearly couldn't control himself, he shouldn't order it anymore. From there, he'd enter a phase of restricting takeout—that is, until he decided he'd just go for it one more time. Rinse and repeat.

However, in our habituation experiment, we first worked on the underlying belief that the food was unhealthy, aiming to reframe this belief to be in line with the idea that all foods are nourishing. Then, he decided to order his favorites with intention and permission every week indefinitely. When plating his meal, he'd put some of each item on his plate, with permission to get more *after* he'd checked in with his body. He used a real plate instead of eating out of the to-go packages, and he sat down at his table without distraction. After several weeks of working on this, he really noticed a difference in his relationship with Chinese takeout. He was paying attention to his food, noticing sensory specific satiety, enjoying leftovers for many days, and not getting overly full. Regular, consistent, nonjudgmental intake of his vilified food helped him to habituate.

Build a Tasty and Balanced Plate

In addition to desired sensory properties and an all-foods-fit mindset, let's consider how structure and planning are involved in gentle nutrition with an intuitive eating for diabetes approach. Sometimes clients ask me if intuitive eating is just eating whatever you want without any structure. To that, I answer no, because that would not be intuitive! To be intuitive, one needs to be in tune with their own body's operating system and signals. To pay no regard to planning or structuring a meal would be in direct opposition to using intuitive wisdom to guide when and what to eat.

So, what is building a tasty and balanced plate all about? The tasty part should be pretty clear—include foods that taste good to *you* on your plate. Remember: if you like it, eat it; if you don't, leave it. There are so many wonderfully nourishing foods in this world, so there's no point in forcing yourself to eat something you don't care for. I've worked with many clients over the years that have forced down foods just because they deemed them "healthy." If you don't care for green smoothies, kale, or cauliflower "rice," no worries—there are many other ways to get the nutrients that those foods provide!

To build a balanced plate, let's consider the six nutrients needed for survival: macronutrients (carbohydrates, protein, and fat), micronutrients (vitamins and minerals), and water. These nutrients are aptly named. We need large amounts of macronutrients (*macro* means large) and smaller amounts of micronutrients (*micro* means small). We only get calories (food energy) from our macronutrients.

- **Carbohydrates** are an essential source of energy for the body. In fact, we require most of our calorie intake (45 to 65 percent) to come from carbs. All carbohydrates convert to glucose in the body; some convert faster and some slower. Slower-digesting carbs, such as whole grains, may help blood glucose management. In addition, all carbs will digest slower in the presence of fat, protein, and fiber. Carbohydrate-rich foods can be a source of a variety of vitamins and minerals, fiber, prebiotics, and/or resistant starch (more on this later). The glucose that carbs provide is the preferred fuel source of the brain and muscles.

- **Protein** is made up of amino acids. When we digest protein, we break it down into individual amino acids. There are twenty amino acids, nine of which are essential, meaning we have to get them from food. Our body uses amino acids for many things including creating antibodies to keep the immune system strong, repairing muscle tissue, creating new cells, making enzymes and hormones, regulating fluid balance, and more. Many protein-rich foods are also good sources of micro-nutrients, such as B vitamins, iron, and zinc.

- **Dietary fat** is required for the proper digestion, absorption, and transport of fat-soluble vitamins (vitamins A, D, E, and K) and phytochemicals (plant pigments). Fat also adds an important textural property to foods. It adds a smoothness to ice cream and a tenderness to baked goods. In addition, fat slows gastric emptying, which is beneficial for reducing blood sugar spikes. If you build your plate like the image below, you're helping to provide your body with a sustaining source of energy from carbohydrates, proteins, and fats.

- **Micronutrients** are vitamins and minerals. While they don't supply calories, many of them function as cofactors and coenzymes for energy-producing reactions in our bodies, which means that without them, vital metabolic functions can't take place. Eating a rich variety of foods often helps us to ensure that we'll get enough micronutrients because they are often contained in foods that also have macronutrients. For example, pinto beans, a carbohydrate source, also contain many essential micronutrients, including iron, calcium, vitamin C, vitamin B6, and magnesium.

- **Water** is an essential nutrient with many important roles in digestion, absorption, excretion, transport, body temperature regulation, and more. As was mentioned in chapter 3, water intake comes from a variety of sources beyond simply drinking plain water.

The image below provides an example of how you can build a balanced plate including all of the six essential nutrients in the proportions needed for optimal functioning. You can use this visual to build your own plate full of foods you like from each category.

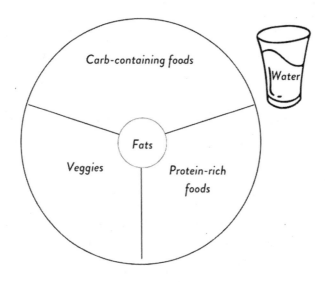

You'll see there are no portion sizes listed here, only proportions. That's because the amount of food needed varies from person to person, and even day to day and meal to meal. For example, two people of the same size and build might plug their metrics into an equation to estimate calorie requirements and come out with the same needs. However, these equations don't take various factors into account that can greatly impact appetite and hunger level, such as sleep, menstrual cycle, illness, stress, mood, and periodic growth spurts (in children). In addition, physical activity may vary for an individual and cause increased hunger either the day of or after a more strenuous level of exertion. For that reason, using your intuitive eating skills in connection with the knowledge of the food groups needed for a meal can lead you to build a plate that is right for your needs.

Also, keep in mind the plate here is meant to represent a meal. Depending on your age, sex assigned at birth, activity level, and medical conditions, you may need to fill your plate more or less. Growing teens, most adults, or those who are highly active (more than sixty minutes of activity per day) will need to fill at least a standard ten-inch dinner plate.

Young children, post-menopausal women, older men, and those who are less active may need to fill a smaller, six-inch salad-size plate. Ultimately, only you know how much food you need. Honor your hunger by giving yourself full permission to adjust your food intake based on feedback from your body. Most people will need three meals plus several snacks daily to meet their needs.

Finally, if you aren't able to eat a balanced plate and keep your blood glucose in range, it's highly likely that you need more medication rather than less food. This is especially true if you weren't eating enough before. Talk to your health care team if this is the case for you.

Use the following food category lists to build your own meals. These lists aren't all-inclusive but will hopefully provide you with some ideas. Note that protein sources marked with a double asterisk (**) will work for both vegetarians and vegans alike; those marked with a single asterisk (*) will work for lacto-ovo vegetarians. If you're a pescatarian, add in fish and seafood as you wish.

- **Carbohydrate sources:** rice, pasta, noodles, bread, biscuits, muffins, bagels, challah, fry bread, hamburger or hot dog buns, English muffins, tortillas, crackers, graham crackers, popcorn, chips, pretzels, quinoa, couscous, bulgur, barley, buckwheat, kamut, spelt, sorghum, wheat berries, farro, millet, kasha, amaranth, freekeh, pita, naan, chapati, roti, cereal, oatmeal, grits, milk, yogurt, granola, waffles, pancakes, legumes (beans, lentils), all fruits and fruit juice, French fries, jelly/jam, honey, sugar, sweets/desserts, certain sauces/condiments, starchy veggies: corn, peas, butternut squash, acorn squash, potatoes, yams, cassava, dasheen, plantain, parsnips

- **Protein sources:** meat, poultry, seafood, eggs*, yogurt*, cottage cheese*, milk*, cheese*, legumes**, nuts**, nut butters**, seeds**, tofu**, tempeh**, edamame**, nutritional yeast**, seitan (wheat protein)**, hemp hearts**, oat bran**, quinoa**, veggie burger**, meat alternative products** such as Impossible or Gardein

- **Fat sources:** oils, butter, ghee, lard, avocado, olives, nuts, seeds, nut butters, dressings, hummus, pesto, cheese, mayonnaise, sour cream, cream cheese, cream, whole cow's milk

- **Veggies:** any type—cooked, raw, as an ingredient in a sauce, stew, soup, smoothie, or juice.

- **Water:** flat or sparkling water, hot or cold unsweetened tea, coffee, milk

One other note: Vegetarians and vegans do need to pay some extra attention to a few key nutrients, specifically: protein, calcium, vitamin D, omega 3, iron, zinc, vitamin B12. If you're in either of these categories, I'd recommend taking a well-rounded multivitamin and mineral supplement, and supplementing single additional nutrients as needed. I'll discuss this more in chapter 5 where dietary supplements will be covered in detail.

Below are examples of balanced meals. See if you can come up with some of your own as well, based on the foods you typically like to eat. The meals below are only examples—they don't represent foods you *must* eat. The options for building a balanced plate are endless, so get creative!

- **Avocado toast:** Sourdough toast spread with avocado and topped with eggs, arugula, and sliced tomato, with hot tea to drink

- **Tacos:** corn tortillas filled with chicken, shredded lettuce, cheese, pico de gallo, and guacamole, with sparkling water to drink

- **Salmon bowl:** rice topped with baked salmon, broccoli roasted with olive oil, and iced tea to drink

- **Pasta:** Spaghetti with meatballs, a side salad with dressing, and lemon water to drink

- **Pad thai:** rice noodles with vegetables, tofu, egg, and chili oil, with water to drink

Cultural Foods

Researchers Willig et al. (2014) and Basinger, Cameron, and Allen (2023) have looked at the intuitive eating practices of people who identify as Black and have T2DM. Many respondents were under the impression that managing diabetes meant restricting foods to "diabetic foods," in addition to having other perceptions of "good" and "bad" foods. The participants also described "rebellious" eating as an emotional response to the burden of a diabetes diagnosis.

It's not surprising that they felt conflicted about what to eat with diabetes, because they were often receiving inappropriate nutrition messages from their own health care providers. In a review by Majeed-Ariss et al. (2015), it was noted that many diverse ethnic groups have experienced being told to "reject culturally traditional foods." Basinger and colleagues outlined the extremely problematic ways in which food discussions took place among culturally diverse individuals with diabetes. These individuals are often unfairly and unnecessarily asked to abandon their cultural food practices without regard to the immense historical importance that food has on our quality of life.

Please note that the meal planning plate above is meant to include *all cultural foods.* There is no need to abandon any food when you have diabetes! There are so many wonderfully delicious cuisines from around the globe and all of them fit—even with a diabetes diagnosis.

The first step to building a balanced plate using your cuisine of choice is to understand which food group each of the foods belongs to. For example, in my husband's Nigerian culture, there are often several types of carbohydrate-based foods as part of one meal. One plate might include fufu (made from cassava), jollof rice, and fried plantain. It's totally fine to include multiple carbohydrate sources; one should simply be mindful of the rest of the plate and the typical blood sugar response. Perhaps the rest of the plate will include stew meat and cooked vegetables to round out the meal.

Challenge the Diabetes Police

If you looked at the inclusive list of foods from all food groups above and thought "I can't eat that!" then it's the "diabetes police" talking. It's the part of you that's monitoring the unrealistic and unnecessary food rules you've stacked up over time, inducing guilt when you don't abide by them. As you've learned by now, food rules backfire. Remind yourself that all foods fit, and practice building and eating a balanced plate at least three times per day. Connect with your inner intuitive eater when you're eating to quiet the diabetes police once and for all.

The diabetes police can come from within or from external instruction, and often comes from clinicians. I often hear, "My doctor told me to cut out [fill in the blank]!" I've heard so many diabetes-policing experiences over the years, ranging from being told to lose weight, cut out carbs, cut out white foods, only eat within certain hours of the day, etc. When the diabetes police are loud, the intuitive self gets silenced. For example, after Anya's labs came back showing high levels of cholesterol, her doctor said to cut out a number of foods. Anya had tried this, but was feeling overly hungry, unsatisfied, and preoccupied with her food. I let her know that rather than cutting foods, she could focus on *adding* foods in. There are a number of foods, especially those high in soluble fiber, that when eaten regularly may help to lower cholesterol, especially LDL cholesterol. No need to cut! Our approach can be affirmative and additive, not negative and punitive.

Many years ago, I worked with a client who had diabetes in addition to several other ailments. She was having trouble keeping her blood sugar in range and had been given a variety of conflicting advice that had left her feeling confused. Much of the advice she'd been given was food-related: cut out this or that. The diabetes police were in full force. In addition to high glucose, she was also having atypical digestive symptoms. She had already tried to limit carbs to control her blood sugar, to no avail.

Based on her symptoms, I suggested a stool test. Turns out, she had an infection with a very tricky bacteria called Clostridium difficile (C. diff) and this was the culprit for her unpredictable blood glucose levels! Once treated, she was able to see an improvement in her levels and she didn't actually need to go on a super-restrictive low-carb diet or cut out food groups at all. For the diabetes police, food is an easy culprit, and it often distracts from other factors at play, such as it did in this case.

REFLECTION

Write or draw a balanced meal that sounds appealing and satisfying to you at this moment. How did you come up with this meal? Are your inner critic or food police saying anything about it? If yes, how might you let some of those thoughts go so that you can truly practice feeding your body, intuitively?

Extra Gentle Nutrition

The remainder of this chapter will discuss some miscellaneous factors that bear on gentle nutrition, particularly when it comes to diabetes care. We'll explore the use of nonnutritive sweeteners, how to understand the glycemic index, and how best to read and use the information on standard nutrition labels.

Nonnutritive Sweeteners

More than a century ago, a brave, imprudent scientist did the unthinkable and tasted a sample from his lab. It tasted sweet! This mystery substance later became known as saccharin and was found to have a very sweet taste (200 to 700 times sweeter than table sugar!); it also contained no calories. Its use became widespread during World War I's sugar shortage and later was marketed as a weight-loss aid and sold as Sweet'N Low, and eventually other trade names: Sweet and Low, Sweet Twin, and Necta Sweet. Since that time, many other nonnutritive sweeteners have taken the stage: acesulfame-potassium, aka Ace-K (Sunett, Sweet One); aspartame (Equal, Sugar Twin); sucralose (Splenda); neotame (Newtame); stevia (Truvia, NutraSweet, Pure Via, Enliten); luo han guo, aka monk fruit (Nectresse, Monk Fruit in the Raw, PureLo); and Advantame.

It's not surprising that people with and without diabetes have taken to using nonnutritive sweeteners, since organizations like the ADA and the American Heart Association (AHA) support their use. But are there any drawbacks? A number of studies to date suggest there could be. In 2023, the WHO released a statement based on the findings of a systematic review that found some potential undesirable effects from long-term use of these sweeteners, such as an increased risk of T2DM, cardiovascular diseases, and mortality in adults (Rios-Leyvraz and Montez 2022). Let me repeat this in case you breezed over it: the review found that T2DM risk may be amplified from using nonnutritive sweeteners! Other studies have found a potential for these sweeteners to increase appetite because they result in less satisfaction in eating, thereby increasing food-seeking behavior; that they may encourage sugar cravings; and that they disrupt gut microbiota composition and function (Yang 2010; Iizuka 2022; Suez et al. 2014).

Nonnutritive sweeteners are often found in sugar-free or reduced sugar drinks, desserts, yogurts, condiments, cereals, snack foods, candies, and gum. If you currently consume these products, it's totally up to you about what you do going forward. Perhaps you feel great consuming them and don't want to stop—this is intuitive eating after all, so you have complete bodily autonomy to decide what works best for you. If you don't currently consume foods or beverages with these sweeteners, perhaps you'll consider some of the controversies outlined in this section, or maybe you'll experiment to see what you think. Just recognize, you don't *have* to use them to control your diabetes, even though the diabetes police might say you do.

The Glycemic Index (GI)

The GI is a numeric score from zero to 100 given to a food based on how quickly it raises blood sugar. All carbs convert to blood glucose, but they do so at different rates. For example, pure glucose—which doesn't occur naturally in foods but is available in tabs or gels and is typically used to treat hypoglycemia—has a GI score of 100, which is the maximum score. All other foods are compared to this maximum. Foods containing fiber or larger amounts of fat tend to have lower GIs. Foods with higher GIs (greater than 70) include bread, potatoes, cereal, rice, and candies. These foods typically cause a peak blood sugar rise about 30 to 45 minutes after consumption. Foods with a moderate GI (45–69) digest more slowly and lead to a peak blood sugar rise at about 60 to 90 minutes after eating. Foods in this category include ice cream, orange juice, cake, and carrots. Foods with a low GI (below 45) cause a more gradual rise in blood glucose that may not peak until several hours later. Low-GI foods include whole grain pasta, milk, yogurt, beans, and chocolate.

The glycemic load (GL) adds another component to the GI by considering the actual amount of carbohydrates consumed. The GL is the GI of the food divided by 100 and multiplied by the amount of available carbohydrates (carbs minus fiber) in grams. Using the meal planning plate and including foods known to slow digestion (foods containing fat, fiber, or protein) is a helpful diabetes management strategy that doesn't require referring to charts or making calculations.

However, if you are someone who manages diabetes with insulin, knowledge of the GI can be helpful in planning when to deliver your insulin bolus. For example, in his book *Think Like a Pancreas* (2020), diabetes specialist Gary Scheiner recommends bolusing well before eating for high-GI foods, bolusing soon before eating for moderate-GI foods, and bolusing after eating or spreading out delivery for low-GI foods or meals that are prolonged or very large. The purpose of this recommendation is to aim to match insulin's peak action with the peak blood glucose rise.

How to Use Nutrition Facts Labels

It's hard to believe that prior to the '90s, packaged foods were not required to carry a nutrition or ingredient label. The Nutrition Labeling and Education Act (NLEA) was passed in 1990 and gave the FDA explicit

authority to require nutrition labeling on most packaged foods. The
first labels began appearing on
packaged foods in 1994 and since
then there have been only slight
adjustments to the labeling requirements (Wartella, Lichtenstein, and
Boon 2010). At right, you'll find an
example of a nutrition label that fits
the requirements as of this book's
publication. In my counseling work,
clients have professed utter confusion regarding nutrition labels,
ingredient lists, and various health
claims on food packaging. Do you
find this confusing as well? Let's
take a moment to clear things up so
that you leave this chapter with a
full understanding of how to interpret the information presented on
packaged food.

Nutrition Facts

5 servings per container

Serving size	1/2 cup (55g)

Amount Per Serving

Calories **200**

	% Daily Value*
Total Fat 10g	13%
Saturated Fat 2g	10%
Trans Fat 0g	
Polyunsaturated Fat 3g	
Monounsaturated Fat 5g	
Cholesterol 0mg	0%
Sodium 250mg	11%
Total Carbohydrate 25g	9%
Dietary Fiber 5g	18%
Total Sugars 10g	
Includes 5g Added Sugars	10%
Sugar Alcohol 0g	
Protein 15g	
Vitamin D 3mcg	15%
Calcium 260mg	20%
Iron 0.9mg	4%
Potassium 705mg	15%

* The % Daily Value (DV) tells you how much a nutrient in a serving of food contributes to a daily diet. 2,000 calories a day is used for general nutrition advice.

Here's how the nutrition facts label breaks down:

- **Servings per container:** How many servings you can expect
  to get out of one package *if* you consume the serving size. For
  the example label, the package supplies 5 servings that are ½
  cup each.

- **Serving size:** Suggested amount to consume; it's the portion
  that the rest of the label is based on. In the example label, the
  serving size is ½ cup or 55 grams (this is the weight of the
  food; since most people aren't weighing their food, this can
  usually be ignored). If you consume 1 cup, then the information in the label must be doubled. Eating intuitively means
  eating the amount you *need*, even if it's more than one serving
  per the label.

- **Calories:** Calories represent the energy we get from food. This product supplies 200 calories per ½ cup portion. Everyone's calorie needs are different.

- **Total fat:** The total amount of fat in one serving, which includes the saturated, trans, polyunsaturated, and monounsaturated fats listed.

- **Percent daily value:** On the right side of the label, you'll see a daily value percentage. This percentage is based on a set daily value that isn't individualized. The daily value uses two thousand calories as its standard and from there calculates estimated requirements for total fat, saturated fat, cholesterol, sodium, total carbohydrate, dietary fiber, added sugars, vitamin D, calcium, iron, and potassium.

- **Cholesterol:** Cholesterol is only present in foods of animal origin. If you have high cholesterol, that refers to the cholesterol in your blood and it doesn't mean you can't eat foods containing cholesterol. There are many factors that impact blood cholesterol levels, and eating foods with cholesterol isn't necessarily it. A 2019 advisory panel revealed there was not a significant association between dietary cholesterol and cardiovascular disease risk (Carson et al. 2020). So, don't worry too much about this number on the label.

- **Sodium:** Sodium comes from salt, which contains sodium chloride. If you've been given a specific sodium recommendation from your health care team, you can use this info to guide your food purchasing decisions and to compare products. Salt is used as a preservative for many foods in addition to being a flavor enhancer. If you're using a packaged food to create a meal, you can offset a high-sodium food by adding some fresh fruits or veggies to the meal.

- **Total carbohydrates:** As a person with diabetes, this is likely the most valuable portion of the label for you, since carbs have a direct impact on blood glucose. Your carb needs are dependent on your energy requirements, age, and physical activity level. On the label, you'll see several categories listed underneath total carbohydrates. **Dietary fiber** is the amount of fiber in one serving size of the food. Humans can't digest fiber into glucose, so you can subtract the amount of fiber listed from the total carbs. Here, it would be twenty-five grams total carb minus five grams fiber equals twenty grams of net carbs. The body will digest twenty grams of carbs from one serving of this food. Listed under dietary fiber is **total sugars**, which includes any naturally occurring sugars (such as lactose in milk products or fructose in fruit products) plus any added sugars (such as honey or table sugar). The amount of **added sugars** is also denoted below the total sugars for those that want to know specifically how much of the total sugars is added, rather than naturally occurring. Last in the list under total carbs is **sugar alcohols.** Sugar alcohols are often added to reduced sugar products, in the form of xylitol, lactitol, mannitol, maltitol, sorbitol, or isomalt. Sugar alcohols are digested much more slowly, require little to no insulin, don't cause sudden glucose spikes, and provide about half the amount of calories when compared to regular sugar. However, excess intake of sugar alcohols can cause bloating and diarrhea.

- **Protein:** Protein needs are highly individual. Most adults need somewhere between 50 and 175 grams each day—that's a huge range! If you're highly active, your needs are on the higher end of that range. If you're more sedentary or have chronic kidney disease, your needs will be on the lower end. Talk to your health care team about your specific needs.

- **Vitamin D, calcium, iron, potassium:** These four micronutrients are listed at the bottom of the nutrition facts label because Americans generally don't get enough of them.

- **Ingredients** (not pictured): Labels will list ingredients in order of descending predominance by weight, meaning the ingredient present in the greatest amount will be listed first with the ingredients in smaller amounts following.

In addition to nutrition labels, some packaged foods will contain health, nutrient, or structure-function claims on the front packaging. Here are some examples that pertain to diabetes:

- **"Sugar Free," "No Sugar," "Zero Sugar":** the product has less than 0.5 grams of sugar per serving, but this doesn't mean it's necessarily carb free! These foods may also contain non-nutritive sweeteners.

- **"No Sugar Added":** there are no sugar ingredients in the food; however, there may be nonnutritive sweeteners and the food may still contain carbs.

Moving Forward

In this chapter, you've been introduced to pillar three of intuitive eating for diabetes: gentle nutrition. I hope you've been able to do some personal exploration and that you leave this chapter with a better understanding of how you can use nutrition inclusively and gently to build balanced, satisfying, and nourishing meals that work for you. In the next chapter, we'll move on to pillar four to discuss your individualized treatment plan.

CHAPTER 5

Pillar Four: Your Individualized Treatment Plan

Your fourth pillar of *Intuitive Eating for Diabetes* is all about your individualized treatment plan. So, what is a treatment plan? A treatment plan is something that emerges after a holistic assessment of your lifestyle, family history, diagnosed health conditions, diagnostic tests, and your personal values. It also takes your culture, environment, and socioeconomic factors into account.

Because there are so many variables that go into making a treatment plan, diabetes treatment plans may vary greatly from one person to the next. Your treatment plan may include prescription medications; dietary supplements; assistive or supportive devices (such as mobility aids or a CPAP for sleep apnea); additional services (such as physical therapy or psychological counseling); and more. Your plan should also continuously evolve to suit your needs.

How would you describe your current treatment plan? Perhaps you aren't certain what your treatment plan entails, or feel it needs a major revision. Maybe you can relate to Ryan, a client I recently worked with, who wasn't quite sure of his diagnosis, what his medications were for, or what types of foods impact blood glucose. Ryan was certainly disconnected from his treatment plan. To help him get reconnected to his plan and his body's needs, we started by reviewing his recent lab results and med list, checked his diabetes knowledge, and discussed what was important to him in terms of values and goals. From there, we were able to chart a path forward.

A 2007 study found that the average primary care visit lasts just seventeen minutes (Tai-Seale, McGuire, and Zhang 2007). With such a short amount of face-to-face time with a provider, it's no surprise that people like Ryan feel unsure of many aspects of their own health despite receiving regular medical care. Imagine how it would feel to be truly armed with knowledge and ready to advocate for your needs at your next medical visit. This chapter is full of information that you can take to your health care team to aid in creating a unique treatment plan that you understand and that truly suits your needs. Your clinician may know a lot about diabetes, but you know your body best—treatment decisions should be made with you on the team.

In this chapter, you'll learn about lab testing, such as how to interpret your results, factors that impact accuracy of results, and how often to test. We'll also dive into important things to know about the classes of diabetes medications on the market, including how they work and potential side effects. You'll also learn about commonly used dietary supplements, including the evidence base surrounding their use, and how to choose a safe, high-quality product if you choose to use them. A discussion of dietary supplement safety, interactions, third-party certification, where to purchase, efficacy, and what to look for will be detailed. By the end of this chapter, expect to understand lab testing, medication options, and supplements in a way that can help you effectively discuss the development of your personalized plan with your treatment team.

Your Holistic Assessment

I invite you to answer the questions below. You can use your companion journal or download the assessment form available to you on : https://www .IntuitiveEatingForDiabetes.com/resources. You'll find a sample holistic assessment available there as well. If some of these questions don't pertain to you or you don't know the information, that's okay—just do your best.

- What medical or mental health diagnoses do you have?

- What medications do you currently take? Include dosages and your reason for using the medication. (Example: Metformin, 500 mg twice daily, for diabetes)

- Have you ever had an adverse reaction to a medication?

- When did you last have lab work done? What was your HbA1c and fasting glucose result? Was anything flagged as out of range?

- If you self-monitor your glucose, whether through a CGM or fingersticks, what is your recent blood sugar range (high and low)?

- How often (if ever) do you experience hypoglycemia (blood sugar under 70)?

- Do you take any dietary supplements, such as vitamins, minerals, or herbs? What is the purpose behind each supplement you take?

- What factors influence your personal diabetes management? What is supportive and what interferes?

- What are your personal goals related to your health and well-being?

Having these holistic assessment notes handy will prove a helpful companion as you move through this chapter and may also be useful to have with you at medical visits.

Lab Testing

Your health care team likely asks you to have lab tests done at least once yearly. When you are changing a medication regimen or monitoring a result more closely, your provider may request blood tests more often, sometimes up to four times per year.

When I meet with clients one-on-one, most of the time they tell me they don't really understand their lab results. Let's go over these lab tests so that you have a better understanding of what the results indicate.

- **Complete blood count** (CBC): This is a group of tests that includes red and white blood cells, hemoglobin, hematocrit, and a number of other tests that help to evaluate whether any anemias or abnormalities within the cells are present.

- **Comprehensive metabolic panel** (CMP, aka chemistry screen): This is a group of tests that includes glucose, electrolytes (potassium, sodium, chloride), and tests that evaluate liver (AST, ALT, bilirubin, alkaline phosphatase) and kidney (BUN, creatinine) function.

- **Lipid panel:** This panel typically tests four types of cholesterol (total cholesterol, VLDL, LDL, and HDL) in addition to triglycerides. Cholesterol is a waxy substance found in your blood. It's made by your liver and also ingested when you eat certain foods. As previously mentioned, the amount of cholesterol in your blood is impacted by many factors. *Total cholesterol* represents the combination of VLDL, LDL, and HDL cholesterol levels. *LDL* stands for low-density lipoprotein. You might think of it as "lousy"; like a train going the wrong direction and dropping hazards off along the way, it heads from the liver out to the rest of the body and drops off cholesterol as it goes, contributing to increased cardiovascular risk. *HDL* stands for high-density lipoprotein and is known as the "healthy" cholesterol. It's like the cleanup crew, picking up the hazards (cholesterol) left by the LDL and taking them back to the train station (the liver). Higher HDL is protective and is associated with decreased cardiovascular risk. *VLDL* stands for very low-density lipoprotein and should be present in low amounts in fasting blood samples. Finally, *triglycerides* are a type of fat. There are many factors that may influence levels, but high levels may be associated with high blood sugar, high alcohol intake, liver or kidney disease, certain medications, inflammation, smoking, thyroid disease, and physical inactivity.

- **Thyroid panel:** A thyroid panel will often include TSH (thyroid stimulating hormone), T3, T4, and thyroid antibodies. These tests aim to determine if your thyroid is working as expected. The thyroid is a gland that produces hormones that influence several body systems. The pituitary gland makes TSH, which then travels to your thyroid and stimulates it to produce the hormones T3 and T4. It's important to test thyroid function because an improperly functioning thyroid can have many ramifications, including negative diabetes health outcomes.

- **Micronutrients:** Vitamins and minerals are necessary for the optimal functioning of body systems. Some that may be tested in routine screenings include magnesium, phosphorus, zinc, vitamin B12, vitamin D, and iron. Unless the micronutrient is stored in the body, like vitamin D or iron (stored as ferritin), it's not always easy to get a great reflection of micronutrient status from a blood test. Another way to determine whether you are getting enough of a particular nutrient is an assessment with a registered dietitian, who can take your health history, medication and supplement usage, activity level, and food intake into account when determining whether you are getting enough.

- **HbA1c:** You're likely very familiar with this test, which is a reflection of your blood sugar over the past 2 to 3 months. Hemoglobin is the iron-containing oxygen transport protein in red blood cells. Ninety-seven percent of normal hemoglobin is made up of four protein chains. A small fraction of the remaining 3 percent is made up of a hemoglobin component called A1c. The rate of A1c formation is directly related to the average concentration of glucose. Thus, when your blood

WHEN HBA1C RESULTS ARE MISLEADING

While HbA1c is considered the gold standard for the diagnosis of diabetes and the assessment of glycemic control, there are numerous conditions that impact its clinical relevance. Conditions that change the life span of red blood cells directly impact the accuracy of HbA1c results. This could include a recent blood loss, sickle cell, use of erythropoietin, kidney failure, hemodialysis, a blood transfusion, iron-deficiency anemia, or liver disease. In addition, if you're of African, Mediterranean, or Southeast Asian descent or have family members with sickle cell anemia or thalassemia, an HbA1c test could be unreliable for diagnosing or monitoring glycemia (NIDDK [National Institute of Diabetes and Digestive and Kidney Diseases] 2018). Some people from these regions have a hemoglobin variant that can interfere with some HbA1c tests. Most people with a hemoglobin variant have no symptoms and may not know that they carry this type of hemoglobin.

If your HbA1c and blood glucose results don't quite add up, you have one of the conditions mentioned above, or think you may have a hemoglobin variant based on your ethnic background, you might want to ask your health practitioner to do further testing. Testing fructosamine instead of HbA1c or using a CGM could provide a more accurate picture of your state of glucose control.

sugars are higher, there is more A1c formed, making it an excellent marker of glycemic control. Since your body makes a whole new set of red blood cells every 120 days, this test is able to provide you with an estimate of your blood sugar over that time frame. If you have diabetes, you've likely been told to aim for an HbA1c of less than 7 percent. For people without diabetes, we expect this level to be less than 5.7 percent. Higher HbA1c levels represent higher average blood sugar over a three-month time period.

- **Fructosamine:** This test reflects a person's average blood sugar level over two to three weeks. Since it doesn't use hemoglobin to estimate the average glucose level, this test is preferred when hemoglobin levels are out of range or in the case of certain blood disorders, such as sickle cell or other hemoglobin variations. In addition, this test may be helpful in assessing more recent blood sugar changes, since it reflects weeks rather than the months that the HbA1c reflects.

- **Urinalysis:** Urine testing will assess things like the pH and color of your urine, in addition to determining whether there is bacteria, glucose, or protein present. Glucose will spill into the urine when blood sugars are running high. Protein in the urine is a sign of early kidney disease.

REFLECTION

If available, look over your most recent lab tests. Was anything marked as out of range? If so, make a note to discuss those results with your provider (if you haven't already). Were any of the tests listed above not performed? If so, perhaps you'll want to make a note to discuss additional testing with your provider.

Considerations Specific to Medications

Some drugs are known to be associated with hyper- or hypoglycemia and some even seem to increase diabetes risk in those without diabetes. These include certain types of antibiotics used to treat UTIs and pneumonia; some types of atypical antipsychotics used to treat schizophrenia or other mental illness; corticosteroids (as mentioned in chapter 1); calcineurin inhibitors used to treat autoimmune conditions; protease inhibitors used in the treatment of viral illnesses; and decongestants (Chou et al. 2013). In addition, many medications prescribed to manage blood pressure and cholesterol negatively impact blood glucose, such as thiazide and thiazide-like diuretics, niacin, statins, and beta-blockers (Goldie et al. 2016; Crandall et al. 2017).

When it comes to prescription medications for diabetes, doctors will often tell patients with elevated sugars to try "diet and exercise" for three months first; I also often hear from clients that they want to avoid medications at all costs. Ultimately, *Intuitive Eating for Diabetes* aims to improve your relationship with food, stabilize your eating patterns, reduce glucose swings, and even lead you to eat a greater variety of nourishing foods, but blood sugar results will vary. Sugars could increase, decrease, or stay relatively the same, depending on what your eating patterns were like before working to eat intuitively. For that matter, if you find that you are eating with attunement yet your blood glucose isn't in range, then it's time for a chat with your health care team. If your glucose and HbA1c are out of ideal range, it's possible that you may need to start (or add more) medication. The good news is that there are many options for meds at this point, and while all medications have the potential for side effects, there may also be the potential for enhanced health outcomes and enhanced food freedoms as well.

In the past several decades, many new diabetes medications and classes of medications have entered the marketplace at rapid speed. Before insulin was discovered in 1921, people with diabetes were treated largely through various extremely restrictive diets or other untested herbs, chemicals, or drugs. Fortunately, extreme carbohydrate restriction proved unnecessary when insulin became available. It wasn't until 1955 that the first oral medication, a class of medications called sulfonylureas, became available. The next oral medication, metformin, in the class of medications called biguanides, was not available in the US until 1995, despite being introduced in Europe in 1957. These medications—insulin, the biguanide metformin, and sulfonylureas—were the only three classes of medications available to treat diabetes until the early 1990s (Mudaliar 2023). In the decades that followed, several new classes of medications became available for use.

Lately, it seems some diabetes medications have taken on a whole new life in the spotlight, with med spa giveaways, feature news stories, and catchy commercials that I even hear my kids randomly singing. Some of these meds have caught the attention of people without diabetes too, specifically the medications that lead to weight loss. This has led to supply chain shortages, fake products, and the manufacturing of products in short supply by compounding pharmacies. This is a problem because compounded meds aren't FDA approved or evaluated for safety, quality, or effectiveness and there have been severe adverse reactions reported.

If you are discussing medications with your clinician, here are some topics you may want to cover in your conversation:

- **Cost:** Is the medication available in generic form? If not, it may have a hefty price tag. Although some brands offer vouchers to ease the financial burden of their med, some medication price tags can leave many individuals priced out.

- **Potential side effects:** There are some diabetes meds that have long track records of success and safety (metformin) and some that have black box warnings (TZDs and GLP-1s). Discuss any risks with your clinician.

- **Expected benefits:** You'll want to weigh the financial cost and potential side effects against the expected benefits the med may offer.

- **How to take it:** Some diabetes meds are injections, while others are pills taken before meals. You'll want to evaluate if you'll be able to take the medication as recommended with your current lifestyle.

In the next several pages, you'll find a brief overview of the most common diabetes medications on the market in the US today (ADA 2023). This isn't an all-inclusive review by any means. What I hope is that you are able to glean some insight into the depth of treatment options available to people with diabetes. The field has come a long way and new research continues to uncover more insights. The future is bright for diabetes treatment. For the most up-to-date medications available, you can always consult the ADA *Standards of Care in Diabetes*, which is available to the public and updated yearly.

Medication Class: Insulin

Before insulin was discovered, a diabetes diagnosis was a death sentence. Fortunately, that is no longer the case! Today, there are a number of different types of insulin on the market that can be used to match the individual's needs. My clients with T2DM often share their wishes to never go on insulin or feeling personally responsible if they do eventually need to use insulin. Listen up: the need to use insulin isn't a personal failing! T2DM is often progressive, meaning that you'll likely need more treatment years down the road than when first diagnosed. Staying in glycemic control will help you live more quality years of life—if insulin can help you do that, then all the gratitude toward insulin!

HOW INSULIN WORKS

As discussed in chapter 1, when the pancreas is fully functional, insulin is released in response to a blood glucose increase and allows the cells to receive glucose for energy. If you are someone that injects insulin to manage your diabetes, your pancreas isn't releasing enough (or any) insulin. There are now many types of insulin available and will be prescribed in accordance with whether you're still making any insulin, how you deliver insulin to yourself (needle and syringe, pen, or pump), your blood sugar levels, your lifestyle, ease of use, and safety considerations. For example, insulin pump users typically only use rapid-acting insulin, while someone who needs a simpler insulin therapy may be prescribed a pre-mixed combination insulin delivered through an auto-injector. This review of medications is to help you feel informed about your diabetes care. Please, never alter your medication regimen without the help and agreement of your clinician.

TYPES OF INSULIN

Insulin has come a long way since it was first prescribed for use. There are now several classes of insulin that can be used to meet the specific needs of the individual. For example, rapid-acting (lispro, aspart, glulisine) and short-acting (regular) insulin are designed to be used with meals because they begin working within 5 to 15 minutes and 30 to 60 minutes, respectively. Regular insulin is a human insulin that has a delayed action time, which means there is a need to inject and then wait about thirty minutes to eat. The benefit of rapid-acting synthetic human insulin is the speed with which it begins working. This quick action time means there is no need to wait to eat after injecting.

Intermediate acting (neutral protamine hagedorn, or NPH) insulin has a slower action time and delayed peak, which may make it less ideal for managing blood sugar in some situations. Long-acting insulin (detemir, glargine) is meant to cover background needs in the way that a fully functioning pancreas does, which is to secrete small amounts of insulin outside of mealtimes to keep blood sugar levels in check.

In addition to the insulin types described, there are also pre-mixed preparations available, such as 70/30, which has a combination of intermediate and rapid- or short-acting insulin together in one injection. Premixed insulin may be helpful for people who need a less complicated insulin prescription, but it may be harder to achieve glucose targets because of the lack of precision with this type of regimen.

All of the insulin types described thus far are given by injection; however there is one type of insulin that has been FDA approved since 2014 that works through inhalation, which is known by the brand name Afrezza. It shares the same potential side effect of hypoglycemia that exists among all insulin preparations; because it's inhaled, it's also associated with throat irritation and cough, and isn't appropriate for use in those who smoke or who have lung disease.

Medication Class: Sulfonylureas

Sulfonylureas are a class of medications that include glyburide (DiaBeta, Glynase PresTab), glipizide (Glucotrol, Glucotrol XL), and glimepiride (Amaryl). They work by directly stimulating the release of insulin from the pancreatic beta cells; thus, they only work in people who are still capable of producing insulin. Because the med stimulates insulin response, they must be taken with a meal that includes carbohydrates to avoid the risk of low blood sugar. In addition, some people experience weight gain, which is a natural side effect of absorbing more nutrition and better glucose control. Sulfonylureas are low cost and may reduce HbA1c by 1 to 2 percent.

Medication Class: Biguanides

Biguanides are oral diabetes medications that work to lower glucose in two ways: first, by increasing glucose absorption, and second, by decreasing glucose output from the liver. Meds in this category include metformin (Glucophage), which is also available in extended release (XR) and liquid formulations (Riomet). This is a commonly used first-line medication with many advantages including its low cost and long track record of safety–it's been FDA approved since 1994. It's also authorized for use in pregnancy and in children ages ten and up. It may reduce HbA1c by one to two percent.

Metformin is generally well tolerated, but some people do experience gastrointestinal side effects such as nausea and diarrhea. Side effects can be lessened by taking the med with adequate food and gradually increasing dosage or using the XR version. Metformin usage may lead to vitamin B12 deficiency, so if you're using metformin you should supplement with a sublingual or chewable vitamin B12 (Berchtold et al. 1969). The ADA recommends regular monitoring of B12 levels if you use metformin (ADA 2017). Metformin is excreted by the kidneys, so your doctor will also need to evaluate your renal function before and during use.

Diabetes and Weight Loss Medications

There are a number of diabetes drugs on the market that may lead to weight loss and are often prescribed *because* they could lead to weight loss. Perhaps you are taking or have considered taking one of these medications. The information I'll present here isn't meant to steer you in one way or another, and I'm not advising or recommending for or against any medication. Medication decisions should be discussed with your medical practitioner. What I do hope to offer here is information that you can use to guide your conversations and make informed decisions.

MEDICATION CLASS: GLUCAGON-LIKE PEPTIDE RECEPTOR AGONISTS (GLP-1 RA)

As of the writing of this book, the GLP-1 RA drugs known as semaglutides are in the spotlight. There are currently three FDA-approved semaglutide products—Ozempic, Rybelsus, and Wegovy—along with a similar medication called Mounjaro, which will be discussed in the next section. Wegovy is a higher-dosage version of the drug, specifically geared toward weight loss for those age twelve and up with "obesity" or "overweight with weight-related medical problems," and is not an approved T2DM treatment. Other GLP-1 RA products include exenatide (Byetta), exenatide XR (Bydureon), liraglutide (Victoza), and dulaglutide (Trulicity).

All of these meds (other than Rybelsus, which is an oral tablet) are injected anywhere from twice daily to once weekly. These drugs act to lower blood sugar and induce weight loss in a number of ways, including stimulating insulin secretion after eating, slowing digestion of food in the stomach (aka delayed gastric emptying), and inhibiting the release of stored glucose (glycogen) from the muscle and liver cells if blood sugar is already high (Collins and Costello 2024). In sum, this leads to more insulin, less glucose, and slower food digestion. Those taking the drug report less hunger and longer satiety due to the drug's effect of slowing digestion. And for many, this means they eat less.

While you might be thinking that less hunger and lower blood sugar sounds great, there are many potential drawbacks to these meds as well. For one, the FDA has issued a boxed warning, or black box warning, for potential increased risk of thyroid c-cell tumors, which was found in animal testing. A boxed warning is the most serious warning from the FDA. Other adverse events reported include nausea, vomiting, weight loss, constipation, diarrhea, low blood sugar, and loss of appetite. These side effects might be lessened by eating enough food and gradually increasing the dosage. In addition, dizziness, mild tachycardia (elevated heart rate), infections, headaches, dyspepsia, and skin irritation at the injection site occur in some people. Some patients taking this medication report nausea and vomiting after eating any more than a toddler-sized food portion, hair loss due to rapid weight loss, and rebound weight gain. Severe potential side effects that warrant immediate discontinuation of the medication include acute pancreatitis, acute kidney injury, and intestinal blockage (ileus).

In addition, these GLP-1 agonists cannot be taken during pregnancy, so women of childbearing age are advised to use contraception. Further, this medication leads to complications when used by people with kidney disease, gastrointestinal disease, or any history of pancreatitis. There is concern over the long-term effects of these medications on the thyroid as well. Plus, without insurance coverage, the drugs are extremely expensive, with some patients reporting a cost of $1400 per month (Ellis 2023).

The positives of these meds include their ability to be used as a first-line medication, to reduce HbA1c up to 1.6 percent, and to reduce cardiovascular risk regardless of HbA1c change. Of course, the side effect associated with use of these drugs that is most talked about is the weight loss (although it's only 4 to 6 percent). Despite the potential for weight loss and metabolic improvements, patients who have used and then discontinued use of the medication have reported immediate weight regain. This was confirmed by a 2022 study that found that one year following the discontinuation of once-weekly semaglutide, participants regained two-thirds of their prior weight loss, and any positive cardiovascular or metabolic changes while on the medication were also lost (Wilding et al. 2022).

MEDICATION CLASS: GLP-1 & GIP (GLUCOSE-DEPENDENT INSULINOTROPIC POLYPEPTIDE) RECEPTOR AGONISTS

Tirzepatide (Mounjaro) is both a GLP-1 and GIP receptor agonist, which means it activates two types of receptors that lead to some of the same effects noted above—enhanced insulin secretion, insulin sensitivity, and delayed gastric emptying. In clinical trials, Mounjaro was found to lower HbA1c by about 1.8 to 2.4 percent, and at the max dosage weight loss was 7 to 13 percent. Mounjaro hasn't been determined to provide the cardiovascular health benefits seen with some of the GLP-1 RA's and has more reported side effects, including a boxed warning for thyroid c-cell tumors. In addition, the gastrointestinal side effects may be more severe, and the med isn't recommended for use in those with any history of gastroparesis. The most common adverse effects reported in clinical trials were decreased appetite, vomiting, constipation, dyspepsia, and abdominal pain. Mounjaro is taken as a once-weekly injection.

MEDICATION CLASS: SODIUM-GLUCOSE COTRANSPORTER-2 (SGLT-2) INHIBITORS

SLGT-2 inhibitors include canagliflozin (Invokana), dapagliflozin (Farxiga), empagliflozin (Jardiance), ertugliflozin (Steglatro), and bexagliflozin (Brenzavvy). These medications are approved for use in those aged ten and older. They work by decreasing glucose reabsorption in the kidneys and have been found to lower HbA1c by 0.6 to 1.5 percent. In addition, they may slow chronic kidney disease (CKD) progression and reduce cardiovascular risk regardless of HbA1c change. Potential side effects include hypotension, UTIs, genital infections, increased urination, weight loss, and ketoacidosis.

MEDICATION CLASS: DIPEPTIDYL PEPTIDASE-4 (DPP-4) INHIBITORS

DPP-4 inhibitors include linagliptin (Tradjenta), sitagliptin (Januvia), and alogliptin (Nesina). These meds act as incretin enhancers to prolong the action of gut hormones, increase insulin secretion, and delay gastric emptying. Potential side effects include headache and flu-like symptoms. In some cases, severe disabling joint pain has been reported. If this happens, stop the med and contact your doctor right away. Pancreatitis has also been reported in clinical trials, and thus, anyone with a history of pancreatitis should avoid this class of medications. Alogliptin can increase risk of heart failure—notify your doctor if you experience shortness of breath, edema, or weakness. DPP-4 inhibitors may decrease HbA1c by 0.6 to 0.8 percent.

MEDICATION CLASS: THIAZOLIDINEDIONES (TZDS)

TZDs work by increasing insulin sensitivity and include the medications pioglitazone (Actos) and rosiglitazone (Avandia). Potential side effects include weight gain, edema, osteoporosis, fractures, and liver toxicity. There are multiple black box warnings for TZD medications (bladder cancer, congestive heart failure, and myocardial ischemia). These meds may lower HbA1c by 0.5 to 1 percent.

As you can see, there are many classes of diabetes medications—and I didn't even cover all of them! Your diabetes treatment will benefit from using your intuitive wisdom in combination with your clinical history and your clinician's advice to come up with strategies that will benefit your diabetes care.

REFLECTION

What medications, if any, do you currently take? What has your experience with diabetes medication been like? Is there anything about your medication regimen that you'd like to review with your diabetes team at your next visit?

Dietary Supplements

According to the FDA, "dietary supplements are intended to add or supplement the diet and are different from conventional food" (FDA 2022). Supplements come in many forms: tablets, capsules, soft gels, gel caps, powders, bars, gummies, and liquids. Commonly ingested supplements include vitamins, minerals, botanicals, herbs, amino acids, and probiotics. The National Health and Nutrition Examination Survey (NHANES) has found a steadily increasing trend in dietary supplement usage since they began collecting data in 1971. According to their assessments, more than half of US adults take at least one supplement (Gahche et al. 2018). Various other reports have surveyed the supplement use of people with diabetes finding that about 22 percent use herbal products and 67 percent use a vitamin or other type of supplement (Shane-McWhorter 2013).

Studies have shown that low intake and/or deficiency in certain nutrients does influence T2DM risk. A comprehensive 2020 review of studies using diverse populations from Asia, Africa, and North America validated the idea that micronutrient deficiencies may lead to oxidative stress and subsequently, insulin resistance and diabetes (Dubey, Thakur, and Chattopadhyay 2020). These nutrients include vitamin A, vitamin E, vitamin C, vitamin D, calcium, magnesium, zinc, potassium, and beta-carotene (Villegas et al. 2009; Fang et al. 2016; Ärnlöv et al. 2009; Vashum et al. 2013; Harding et al. 2008; Ekmekcioglu et al. 2017; Chatterjee et al. 2017; Shah et al. 2018). These and other substances found to benefit those with diabetes are outlined below. For many supplements, use isn't recommended if you are pregnant or breastfeeding, mostly because safety is simply unknown. Always discuss the use of supplements with your health care team.

In the US, the FDA's role is to enforce specific manufacturing and labeling regulations and to inspect facilities, monitor adverse event reports, and remove tainted or misbranded products from the market. Within the FDA, the Federal Trade Commission (FTC) is responsible for acting on any deceptive or unfair marketing practices from supplement companies. Whereas prescription medications are required to receive FDA approval for safety and efficacy through a five-step process that can take many years, dietary supplements aren't required to undergo this scrutinous approval. The Dietary Supplement Health and Education Act (DSHEA) of 1994 established definitions and regulatory laws over dietary supplements. However, the dietary supplement market has grown tremendously since DSHEA was enacted in 1994. Back then, the public internet was only three years old and e-commerce sites such as Amazon were nonexistent. In 1994, the market for dietary supplements was about $4 billion (Crawford et al. 2022). Now, the global supplement market size is nearly $70 billion and is expected to rise to over $160 billion by 2033. The US is responsible for 33.2 percent of the market, or about $22 billion (Future Market Insights 2023).

Over 15 percent of the total supplement market is represented by e-commerce, with Amazon raking in 77 percent of those supplement sales (Brush 2021). Thus, this is an industry that has become harder and harder to regulate, especially when many supplements are purchased through third-party sites, such as Amazon. In fact, this was such an issue that in 2020 Amazon began requiring sellers to provide documentation of quality control and a certificate of product analysis to sell on the platform (French 2023; Amazon n.d.). However, a case series study published in 2022 found that after testing thirty dietary supplements that were purchased from amazon.com in May of 2021, there were problems with nearly 60 percent of them (Crawford et al. 2022). These problems included inaccurate labels, ingredients listed on labels but not detected in analysis, and substances in the product that were not listed on labels. None of these tested products had third-party certification, which will be discussed further below.

So how can a consumer like you utilize dietary supplements but also ensure the safety and efficacy of the products you decide to use? I have a few suggestions for you.

1. **Use only products with third-party certifications.** These are independent and thus unbiased programs that inspect and test raw materials, manufacturing sites, and finished products. In North America, there are dozens of third-party certifiers,

each with their own standards to meet for a product to sport the certifier's seal of approval. Here are some common ones:

- **Certified Gluten-Free:** These products are certified through independent lab testing to contain less than 20 parts per million (ppm) of gluten, which is especially important for people with celiac disease.

- **National Sanitation Foundation (NSF):** NSF-certified products meet strict standards for ingredients used in dietary supplements. Products are evaluated for unacceptable levels of pesticides, herbicides, and contaminants, such as heavy metals like lead and arsenic. Products that are "NSF Certified for Sport" meet additional standards to confirm that they are free of contaminants, masking agents, and over 270 banned substances.

- **US Pharmacopeia (USP):** To wear the USP seal of approval, products must contain all ingredients listed on the label in the potency claimed, be free of contaminants and unlabeled ingredients, and dissolve in a way that the body can actually absorb the active ingredients. The Kirkland brand sold at Costco and the brand Nature Made have many products bearing the USP seal.

2. **Obtain a membership to consumerlab.com.** ConsumerLab is a watchdog organization with a mission to "help consumers and health care professionals find the best quality health and nutrition products through independent testing and evaluation" (ConsumerLab n.d.). It currently costs about $60 per year to join. With membership, you can search the site for product reviews related to health, wellness, and nutrition including herbal products, vitamins, minerals, sport and energy products, health protection devices, and more. ConsumerLab pulls products, tests them, then issues a report for what they've found. This allows consumers to know whether certain products

contain harmful heavy metals, if the ingredients are correctly listed, and includes a price comparison of various brands.

3. **Purchase directly from the brand or a verified health professional's dispensary.** Unfortunately, some third-party e-commerce retailers may sell adulterated supplements or may not store products at optimal temperatures. Amazon is the largest retailer of supplement products. However, the company has come under fire for its lack of due diligence with regard to counterfeit products being sold on its site. In the fall of 2023, the dietary supplement company NOW identified as many as eleven different sham products mimicking the brand's appearance being sold across more than twenty Amazon storefronts (French 2023). Many of these products contained pharmaceuticals and food allergens! To be on the safe side, I recommend purchasing direct from the manufacturer or through a valid professional dispensary, such as Fullscript.

4. **Don't be duped by marketing schemes.** Unfortunately, there was an uptick in "immunity boosting" supplement marketing and unauthorized ads during the COVID-19 pandemic. A Consumer Reports investigation entitled "Beware Dietary Supplements Marketed Online" found that the mass of schemers was just too much for regulators to keep up with, and as a result, vulnerable people not only lost money but also risked their health by taking products with unsubstantiated claims. The new, modern snake-oil salesperson now hides behind robocalls, texts, and spam emails with catchy language that sounds too good to be true—usually because it is (Felton 2021). Even the smartest, most skeptical of us can get tricked when we feel desperate for a solution. It's important to evaluate what you encounter critically.

5. **Always discuss supplement usage with a qualified health professional.** When I meet with clients who are using dietary

supplements, I ask them about the intent behind the products they use. I'm often surprised when I hear that they began taking a product based on the recommendation of an anecdote from a friend or relative, or an untrained salesperson at a vitamin shop or grocery aisle. The perception of a product being "natural" seems to cloud the possibility that the product can also be strong enough to cause harm. Among health professionals, registered dietitians are uniquely skilled at helping individuals make sense of their dietary supplement needs.

Dietary Supplements for Diabetes

If you are planning to take a dietary supplement with the intention of it somehow benefiting your health, there are a few important things to assess before you fork over your cash. First and foremost, is there evidence to support the efficacy of the product? Does the active ingredient interact with any other medications or supplements? Will it cause any side effects? Below, I've highlighted some common supplements and grouped them into categories based on whether there is evidence that use will improve blood glucose control (McKennon 2000).

- **Supplements that may improve blood glucose control:** Aloe, berberine, chromium, cinnamon, turmeric/curcumin, fenugreek, glucomannan, magnesium, milk thistle (silymarin), turmeric/curcumin, vitamin D

- **Supplements that may not improve blood glucose control:** Alpha-lipoic acid, apple cider vinegar (pill), bitter melon, beta-carotene, khat

- **Supplements that need more research to determine effect on blood sugar:** American ginseng, apple cider vinegar (liquid), cassia cinnamon, gymnema sylvestre

- **Supplements that may worsen blood sugar control:** Digestive enzymes, conjugated linoleic acid (CLA), niacin (high dose)

Here's a bit more about supplements that may improve blood glucose control or diabetes-related side effects.

ALPHA LIPOIC ACID (ALA)

ALA is an antioxidant produced naturally in the body and can also be obtained from foods such as red meat, organ meat, spinach, broccoli, potatoes, yams, carrots, beets, and yeast. While it has not been shown to significantly reduce blood sugar levels, taking 600 to 1800 mg daily may improve symptoms of diabetes-related peripheral neuropathy (Hsieh et al. 2023).

ALOE

Aloe is a cactus-like plant that grows in hot, dry climates such as Texas, Florida, and Arizona. You probably know aloe for its cool, soothing impact on sunburned skin when applied topically. Aloe can also be used orally. Oral aloe may help reduce blood glucose and HbA1c for people with diabetes, but it may be most effective in those with a fasting glucose over 200 mg/dL (Budiastutik et al. 2022; Dick, Fletcher, and Shah 2016). The forms (powder, extracts, raw crushed leaves, fresh extracted juice) and dosage (100–1000 mg of powder or 15–150 mL of juice) of aloe tested have varied greatly across studies. Aloe is generally well tolerated when used in these dosages; however aloe latex is associated with a greater risk of side effects.

BERBERINE

Berberine is an alkaloid taken from a variety of plant sources. There is evidence to support its efficacy in lowering glucose, cholesterol, and blood pressure (Yin, Xing, and Ye 2008). Berberine, at a dosage of 500 mg two to three times daily with meals, is associated with reductions in fasting blood glucose, postprandial glucose, and HbA1c. It's been found to be more effective than placebo and just as effective as prescription medications metformin, sulfonylureas, or glitazones (Dong et al. 2012). Berberine should not be used during pregnancy or lactation. The most common side effects are gastrointestinal (diarrhea, constipation, flatulence, abdominal pain, and vomiting). Since berberine lowers glucose, use caution when combining with other glucose-lowering agents. As always, any potential contraindications of use should be reviewed with your doctor or pharmacist.

CHROMIUM

Chromium is an essential mineral that is found naturally in many foods, including meats, grains, fruits, vegetables, nuts, spices, brewer's yeast, beer, and wine (NIH 2022). There appears to be an association between low levels of chromium and impaired glucose (Asbaghi et al. 2020). Chromium has been found to enhance insulin activity, thus reducing levels of insulin resistance, and has been termed a glucose tolerance factor (GTF). Meta-analyses published in 2020 and 2014 found chromium to be effective in reducing HbA1c and fasting glucose in people with diabetes (Asbaghi et al. 2020; Suksomboon, Poolsup, and Yuwanakorn 2014). For diabetes, taking 500 mcg twice daily may lower HbA1c significantly.

CINNAMON

Cinnamon is naturally obtained from the dried inner bark of certain evergreen trees. It's used in many cuisines around the world and is easy to find in most local grocery stores—I'd recommend looking for ceylon cinnamon that has been third-party tested for contamination. Studies evaluating the effectiveness of cinnamon for glucose-lowering have given mixed results. However, recent meta-analyses have shown a significant decrease in fasting blood glucose (Deyno et al. 2019; Zarezadeh et al. 2023). One gram (1,000 mg or 1-2 teaspoons) of cinnamon bark powder may help to lower blood sugar levels in people with T2DM or prediabetes.

FENUGREEK

Fenugreek is an aromatic herb with a taste and aroma similar to maple syrup. It's native to the Mediterranean region, southern Europe, and western

Asia. Its seeds are used as a spice and in traditional medicine, while its leaves are eaten as a vegetable in India. The fenugreek seed seems to improve glucose control in T2DM, according to some studies (Neelakantan et al. 2014; Gong et al. 2016; Hassani et al. 2019). The most effective doses and formulations are powdered seed or debittered seed powder in amounts of 5 to 100 mg daily, taken as capsules or added to meals.

GLUCOMANNAN

Glucomannan is a soluble fiber usually obtained from the konjac plant. It's been used as a food and medicine in Asian cultures for more than a thousand years. Some research points to glucomannan's potential to improve glucose control in people with T2DM. It may also aid in improving cholesterol levels and blood pressure (Zhang et al. 2023). Most clinical research suggests that a dosage between 3 and 15 grams daily is efficacious.

MILK THISTLE

Milk thistle is a plant found in many places around the world with a long history of medicinal use, dating back to ancient Greece. Milk thistle seed extract is up to 80 percent silymarin, which contains the primary active component. In 2020, a meta-analysis reviewing 16 studies with almost 1400 subjects suggested that, in comparison to placebo, milk thistle was able to significantly reduce fasting blood glucose and HbA1c (McKennon 2000). The recommended dosage for this benefit is 200 mg three times per day (Huseini et al. 2006). For best efficacy, look for a product with at least 58 percent silymarin. Milk thistle is generally well tolerated.

MAGNESIUM

Magnesium is an essential mineral involved in metabolism and nervous system functioning. Magnesium can easily be obtained from food, but almost half of the US population doesn't get enough. Low levels may be due to both inadequate intake and poor soil concentrations. In addition, certain conditions, such as diabetes, can deplete magnesium. Magnesium deficiency may even be involved in the development of insulin resistance and T2DM (Pelczyńska, Moszak, and Bogdański 2022). A large meta-analysis found that magnesium intake may be associated with a decreased risk of developing T2DM (Dong et al. 2011). Magnesium is typically found in whole grains, beans, nuts, and green leafy vegetables. Higher magnesium levels and intake in individuals seems to correlate with a reduced risk of diabetes (Fang et al. 2016). Intake of magnesium supplements and fortified foods should be kept under 350 mg, which is the tolerable upper intake level (UL) to avoid potential side effects.

TURMERIC (CURCUMIN)

Turmeric is a rhizome and member of the ginger family with anti-inflammatory properties and a long history of use in Chinese and Ayurvedic medicine. Curcumin is the active component of turmeric. Research supports a positive effect of turmeric use on glycemic values for those without diabetes and in preventing diabetes for those diagnosed with prediabetes (Marton et al. 2021). Turmeric is generally well tolerated and the typical recommended dosage is 1500 mg of curcuminoids taken in two divided doses (Chuengsamarn et al. 2012).

VITAMIN D

The relationship between vitamin D status and diabetes has been of immense interest in the scientific community over at least the past decade. Observational studies have found an association between low blood levels of the vitamin and T2DM risk. A 2022 review of thirteen studies found that vitamin D deficiency was significantly associated with the development of both T1DM and T2DM (Abugoukh et al. 2022). Other studies have found vitamin D insufficiency to be associated with lower levels of insulin release, insulin resistance, and T2DM (Lips et al. 2017). Vitamin D receptors are found on the insulin-secreting beta cells of the pancreas, and vitamin D may protect beta cells from immune attack because of its role in regulating T-cell responses (Marino and Misra 2019). It's a fat-soluble vitamin found naturally in some fish, mushrooms, dairy products, liver, and egg yolks. The body can also create vitamin D in the skin with sun exposure.

There has been much debate about recommended vitamin D dosages over the years. Michael Holick, a leading vitamin D researcher, has suggested that the lab cut offs for what are considered "normal" levels are too low and that the amount of vitamin D needed for optimal health is higher than standard recommendations. If you are a higher body weight, it's also possible that you'll need more vitamin D to attain adequate levels. Therefore, dosages of vitamin D should be determined alongside your health care team after reviewing your personal factors.

REFLECTION

What questions would you like to bring to your doctor about meds, supplements, or labs at your next medical visit?

Moving Forward

We've covered a lot in this chapter. I hope that you feel an increased level of knowledge when it comes to labs, meds, and supplements. Without knowledge, it's hard to advocate for the kind of diabetes care and treatment plan you need. I hope you'll feel prepared, confident, and ready to advocate for yourself the next time you head to a diabetes care appointment. In the next chapter, we'll dive into the important topic of self-advocacy in great detail, and discuss how to partner with your health care team.

PART 2

Creating a Diet-Free Lifestyle That Works for You

CHAPTER 6

Self-Advocacy and Partnering with Your Health Care Team

Your diabetes care team may include doctors, nurses, physician assistants, registered dietitians, therapists, podiatrists, dentists, cardiologists, nephrologists, and other health care professionals. It can be time-consuming, costly, and confusing to have so many team members. Oftentimes appointments feel rushed, and you may be left feeling unheard. In addition, for many people with diabetes, there are serious barriers to receiving and maintaining regular medical care. These barriers may include access to care, stigmatizing treatment, burnout, and financial constraints. Lack of health care coverage and low use of health care services is associated with poor glycemic control (Zhang et al. 2012). This chapter will cover how to access the health care you need, find team members that are a good fit, make the most out of appointments, and advocate for your needs.

Before you dive in, I invite you to take a minute to consider how you currently feel about your health care team and your diabetes treatment overall. Jot down any thoughts you have about this topic in your companion journal.

Advocate for Weight-Inclusive Care

I hope that by now you are fully aware of the benefits of weight-inclusive care. However, perhaps you're now stuck wondering how to get your clinicians on board with this approach. Maybe you're thinking you don't want to be a pain, and so you'll just consider putting up with the weight-focused treatment you've been getting. But the thing is, when clinicians are focused on weight, they miss things. Here's an example: Rebecca Hiles, who shared her experience of weight stigma–fueled medical neglect on *Good Morning America* and in *Cosmopolitan* magazine in 2019, was told over and over to simply lose weight when she reported breathing problems to her clinicians (Dusenbery 2018). For six years she was told that her troubled breathing was due to her weight, but when a new doctor finally did a thorough evaluation, it was determined that she actually had lung cancer. This delayed diagnosis of her life-threatening condition led to the eventual removal of her entire left lung.

Unfortunately, weight bias appears to be rampant in the medical field. Aubrey Gordon—fat activist, podcast host, and author—has shared her personal experiences with medical weight bias and anti-fat sentiment, first via the pseudonym @yrfatfriend and then in her book, *What We Don't Talk About When We Talk About Fat* (2020). She described an urgent care visit where her blood pressure was retaken multiple times because the nurse was so shocked that someone of her size could have "normal" blood pressure. The nurse even commented, "obese patients don't have good blood pressure" (141).

Negative health care experiences like these often lead to health care avoidance. Studies show that higher-weight women are less likely than thinner women to seek health care (Mensinger, Tylka, and Calamari 2018). Regrettably, experiences of medical weight bias and anti-fat sentiment seem to be commonplace. A 2014 study found that 53 percent of women and 38 percent of men reported being shamed by a physician, with weight as one of the top reasons for the experience (Darby, Henniger, and Harris 2014). Other studies have found similar results. Puhl and Brownell (2006) surveyed over 2000 study participants with BMIs in the "overweight" and "obese" range and asked them about sources of stigma in their life. The participants reported stigma coming from physicians (69 percent), nurses (46 percent), dietitians or nutritionists (37 percent), and mental health professionals (21 percent). Weight bias, which falsely applies negative stereotypes to higher weight people, results in weight stigma. A weight-biased perspective sees people as lazy, lacking willpower, incompetent, unattractive, and to blame for their weight—none of which is true, of course. Weight stigma may include moral discrediting and inappropriate assumptions about the lifestyle or health-related behaviors of higher weight individuals.

While it may seem like weight stigma is just mean and judgmental, it's actually a chronic stressor that may increase cardiometabolic risk on the part of those who experience it (Pearl et al. 2017). When you experience weight stigma, your body releases a stress response that is characterized by a host of bodily actions that can lead to elevated blood pressure and cortisol (Himmelstein, Belsky, and Tomiyama 2014). In addition, the results of a 2015 study found that the perception of weight stigma was strongly associated with poor outcomes in people with T2DM. The study participants had higher hemoglobin HbA1c levels, more diabetes-related distress, and struggled with diabetes self-care, including nutrition, exercise, and glucose testing (Potter et al. 2015). Further evidence has also linked weight stigma to high blood pressure, disordered weight control practices, binge eating, poor body image, clinical eating disorders, low self-esteem, and depression among all age groups (Tylka et al. 2014).

Maybe you can relate to a stigmatizing experience my client, Jackie, recently shared with me. Jackie went to her doctor for a routine checkup and after finding that her blood sugar was *slightly* elevated, her doctor told her to stop eating cake. However, this doctor didn't even ask Jackie about her eating habits; she just made a biased assumption. In fact, Jackie doesn't even like cake! Not to mention that Jackie is in recovery from an eating disorder. Assumptions about how someone eats or moves based on their body size isn't only rude and inappropriate, but also dangerous as it may lead patients to avoid health care to circumvent these uncomfortable and traumatizing interactions. This client's experience is in line with findings from a 2023 study that surveyed internists and endocrinologists and found that they held moderate levels of bias toward individuals with T2DM and even stronger levels of biases for patients with T2DM in larger bodies, assuming their patients were lazy, unmotivated, and non-compliant (Bennett and Puhl 2023).

It's clear that there's a strong need for stigma reduction among physicians and other allied health professionals. Learning how to navigate weight-focused health care will serve as a way to protect your own well-being against the weight bias and stigma that may otherwise affect it. As a patient, you have the right to ask your provider for a visit that's not focused on diet and weight. You could consider calling ahead to ask about the willingness of the practice to offer weight-inclusive care. If you are in a larger body, you may want to inquire about the availability of accessible seating, exam tables, and blood pressure cuffs. If you live in an urban area with many clinics to choose from, shopping around may be an option for you. However, if you live in a more rural area where there are fewer choices when it comes to health care, you may not have many providers to choose from. When you don't have very many options, self-advocacy and boundary setting will be your most valuable tools.

Also keep in mind that it's not just weight that can lead providers to make unhelpful and generalized suggestions. Luis came to me as a 16-year-old varsity basketball player. His doctor had recently done some bloodwork and found that he had a HbA1c of 5.7 percent, which is just 0.1 percent into the prediabetes range. Despite all other labs looking great, the doctor told him to cut out carbs and sugar. As a growing athlete with high calorie needs, Luis was confused, and his parents were very worried since diabetes does run in their family. Luis' parents were unsure of how to feed their thin, athletic teenager after the doctor's remarks. As a result, by the time Luis and his parents met with me, he was undereating and anxious about food. I helped Luis and his family to feel less anxious about the marginally elevated lab result. After our sessions together, they were able to understand how to offer balanced meals and snacks without cutting out any foods.

Navigating Weight-Centric Health Care

Since 2009, writer, activist, speaker, and athlete Ragen Chastain has been sharing the concepts of size acceptance and advocating for weight-inclusive care through her blog, *Dances with Fat*. Her "What to Say at the Doctor's Office" cards have served as a helpful self-advocacy tool for many larger-bodied people experiencing stigma from a doctor. On her blog she describes how she's been prescribed weight loss for a myriad of conditions, including a broken toe and strep throat (Chastain 2013). The cards, which are available in English, Spanish, French, and German, are aimed at helping people communicate their needs for evidence-based and appropriate health care. You can print and hand the cards to the health care provider or use the phrases as a starting point for your own authentic dialogue about your health care needs. Here are some of the helpful phrases that Chastain includes on her cards:

- Please don't weigh me unless it's medically necessary (i.e., for proper medication dosage) and don't tell me the number unless I ask.

- In our limited time together today, I'd like to focus on [what I came in for].

- Do thin people get this health problem? What do you recommend for them?

- The research I've seen shows that the vast majority of people who attempt weight loss fail, and many actually gain weight long term... [Therefore,] please don't prescribe weight loss as a health intervention (Chastain 2013).

I've shared Chastain's tips many times over with patients in my own practice. Many have expressed their anxiety about standing up for their needs or being ignored despite the card. Some find it helpful to bring loved ones along as support to appointments. Others have opted to switch providers.

Alice was putting off scheduling a medical checkup because of the dreaded weigh-in typical of weight-normative clinics. When she learned that she could actually turn down this shaming practice, she was excited and nervous to give it a try. Her health is important to her, and she knew she was doing herself a disservice by avoiding the appointment. Armed with her newfound empowerment, she went in and set some boundaries with the staff and clinicians. She said no thank you when the medical assistant asked her to step on the scale and she let her doctor know right off the bat what she would and would not like to focus on in her visit. Thankfully her requests were honored without resistance, and she left the office feeling proud and capable.

Your Doctor Isn't a Nutrition Expert

In the US and United Kingdom (UK), the majority of medical students receive an average of only eleven hours of nutrition training throughout an *entire* four-year medical education program. Nutrition is insufficiently included in the medical curriculum, regardless of the country, setting, or year of medical school education (Crowley, Ball, and Hiddink 2019). This disparity affects the knowledge, skills, and confidence of future doctors to effectively provide nutrition education to patients like you. The National Academy of Sciences recommends at least twenty-five hours of nutrition content be included in medical education, but as of 2010, only 27 percent of US medical schools met that minimum (Millard 2023). To put this into perspective, consider that an undergraduate general education nutrition class includes approximately forty-five hours of face-to-face instruction. So, if you took a three-unit college nutrition class, you would have received 75 percent more nutrition education than most doctors!

Despite this lack of training in nutrition, primary care guidelines direct physicians to provide nutritional guidance and weight loss interventions to their patients in higher BMI categories, even though they are poorly suited to do so. This leads doctors of higher weight patients to place undue focus—in their already time-constrained visits—on weight rather than the presenting concern of the patient.

A patient-centered, weight-inclusive approach is the most ethical approach for a practitioner to use with you. This is because it considers your best interest, aims to avoid harm, focuses on compassionate care, and holds you in unconditional positive regard. If all clinicians provided weight-inclusive care, it's possible that some aspects of health care would feel more accessible. What would it be like for you to bring this best practice paradigm to the attention of your providers? Are you ready to advocate for yourself and ask for shame-free, weight stigma–free care to potentially improve your health care experience? Maybe you'll be the next seed of change.

REFLECTION

Write down at least one question you'd like to ask or one boundary you'd like to set at your next diabetes-related appointment.

Find Your Team

Despite being one of the richest countries in the world, the US health care system ranks dead last (and has since 2004) when compared to the other ten wealthiest nations (Schneider et al. 2021). While the US spends the most and has the most advanced technology, there are tremendous deficits in access to care, efficiency, equity, and outcomes. Navigating the complex US health care system is a frazzling and frustrating experience for many. America's insurance-based health care system contains a myriad of options: private pay, employer sponsored, Medicare, Medicaid, Veterans Affairs benefits, etc.

The Affordable Care Act

In 2010, the US Congress passed the Patient Protection and Affordable Care Act (ACA). This landmark legislation dramatically improved health care coverage and quality for millions of Americans. With the passage of the ACA, insurers can no longer deny or charge more for health coverage if you have a preexisting condition, such as diabetes. In addition, the ACA allowed millions of Americans to gain health coverage with access to essential health benefits like outpatient care, emergency services, hospitalization, mental/behavioral health treatment, preventive care, prescription drugs, laboratory services, rehabilitative care, and more. To learn more about the ACA and protections for people with diabetes, visit https://diabetes.org/advocacy/know-your-rights/health-insurance-update.

Types of Insurance in the US

In general, there are three types of government-sponsored health plans in the US. Medicaid is the state-administered insurance program for certain individuals and families that meet income limits. Eligibility requirements are state-specific. Medicare is a federal health insurance program for people who are 65 years old or older. You may also qualify for Medicare if you have end-stage renal disease (ESRD) or in certain cases of disability, even if you are under age 65. Lastly, if you are a veteran of the US armed forces, you (and sometimes your family) may be eligible for benefits and services from the Department of Veterans Affairs (VA).

If you don't qualify for Medicaid, Medicare, or VA health insurance and need health coverage, check out the health insurance marketplace at healthcare.gov. It's simply a way for you to shop and compare different private health insurance plans all in one place. If you purchase health insurance through the marketplace and meet certain income requirements, you may qualify for financial assistance to pay for the cost of the plan.

> ## DID YOU KNOW?
>
> All veterans with T2DM who were exposed to herbicides such as Agent Orange during service may be eligible for disability compensation and health care. Contact the VA for an Agent Orange Registry health exam.

Medication Affordability

You've likely experienced the economic burden that having diabetes brings. Even with insurance, diabetes costs add up, with medications and supplies typically accounting for nearly 20 percent of the cost burden (Parker et al. 2024). However, the cost of delaying treatment or short-cutting treatment recommendations can lead to even larger medical bills down the road, not to mention the detriment this brings to health outcomes.

If the cost of caring for your condition is causing anxiety or tempting you to delay or reduce treatment, I'd invite you to speak to your diabetes team about your barriers and concerns. They may have ideas or resources to help you lower costs. Here are some ways that others with diabetes have been able to lower costs:

1. If you're using medication, ask if there's a lower-cost option that may work for you.

2. Ask your provider or pharmacist if they know of any co-pay assistance programs or coupons for the medication you're using to help with out-of-pocket costs. These are often available through pharmaceutical websites or directly from your provider or pharmacist.

3. Inquire about patient assistance programs. Many drug manufacturers, state programs, and nonprofits offer medication

assistance. You can find out more about what you may qualify for by asking your diabetes care team or local pharmacy.

Advocate groups such as the ADA have been working to create partnerships with health organizations and drug manufacturers to increase access to affordable medications. Medicare and some state-regulated health insurance plans have now capped out-of-pocket costs for insulin. You can learn more and stay up to date at https://diabetes.org. There you'll find resources for affordable insulin, community services, health insurance information, and more.

Get the Most Out of Your Appointments

Diabetes care includes self-monitoring, screening exams, and appointments throughout the year. Daily care includes blood sugar checks, foot checks, medication taking, physical activity, and nourishing food intake. If your treatment has changed or you are working to meet a diabetes target, your doctor may want to check your HbA1c and have a clinic visit about every three months. If you're meeting your treatment goals and/or your treatment plan hasn't changed, you'll likely meet with your doctor and have an HbA1c check every six months. It's also recommended to have a dental cleaning every six months. In addition, annual recommendations include a flu shot, kidney and cholesterol tests, a dilated eye exam, hearing check, and a complete foot check (CDC 2023).

While the CDC provides the recommended care schedule detailed above, there may be some discrepancies between recommendations and practice. I've had many patients tell me that their own diabetes care doesn't reflect these guidelines. In fact, my client Aaliyah told me that every time she logged in to her patient portal, she'd get a pop-up message that she was overdue for her foot exam. When she asked her doctor about this at her checkup, she was told to ignore it and ended up leaving the office without this critical exam. So, while it's your physicians' responsibility to do a thorough diabetes assessment each year, it will also fall on you to know what needs to be done and to advocate for the care you need and deserve.

Let's take this foot exam as an example. It's important for individuals to check their own feet daily *and* to have a clinician examine them at least yearly. Why check your feet? Diabetes plus an untreated sore or cut can easily lead to an infection. If you don't check your feet, there could be an infection festering without your knowledge. It's especially easy for you to be unaware of something going on with your feet if you have any kind of nerve damage, which happens to be present in 50 percent of people with diabetes. Nerve damage can take away your ability to feel something going on with your feet. Moral of the story: insist on a foot exam (or any other recommended or routine screening) from your clinician, even if they say you don't need it. (Side note: If you're unable to easily see the bottom of your feet for home checks, try using a mirror or asking a trusted person for help.)

A Letter to Your Health Care Provider

One way to set boundaries and to attempt to get your needs met with health care providers is to provide a letter detailing the kind of care you want and don't want. I've created a sample letter that you are welcome to use with your providers if you'd like; it is available at: https://www.Intuitive EatingForDiabetes.com/resources alongside the rest of the free tools for this book.

Resources for Weight-Inclusive Providers

Does finding a weight-inclusive diabetes provider sound like an elusive dream? A few folks who are passionate about helping others identify health care providers that will provide a weight stigma–free encounter have put together a "Weight-Neutral Providers Lead List" via a Google Doc accessible at the following URL: https://tinyurl.com/weightinclusiveproviderlist. The creators of this list are quick to warn that a name on this list doesn't mean the provider explicitly practices weight-inclusive care, but rather that at least one person during at least one visit didn't experience weight stigma from the listed provider. In addition, https://barehealth.co provides a searchable database of size-inclusive providers in the US. Both sites also allow you to recommend a provider that you've had a positive experience with as an addition to the database.

To find a certified intuitive eating counselor around the globe, you can search the database available at https://www.intuitiveeating.org/certified-counselors. On this list, you'll find a wide range of professionals (dietitians, therapists, health coaches, psychologists, professors, and others) who have successfully completed the standardized training program developed by Evelyn Tribole and Elyse Resch.

If these resources still don't provide you with a lead to a provider open to new patients in your service area, I'd invite you to utilize the other self-advocacy resources outlined in this chapter, namely the letter, the phrases, the boundaries around practices such as weighing, and calling ahead to ask about inclusivity.

Moving Forward

I hope you are feeling prepared and empowered after learning about the ways in which you can access or improve your diabetes care. In the next chapter, "Diabetes Care, Your Way," we'll dig into your personal values and determine how aligned your actions are with your values toward diabetes self-care. We'll discuss why making changes is so hard and how you can make the changes you really want to make *and* stick with them.

CHAPTER 7

Diabetes Care, Your Way

Changing a behavior is tough work, even when the change is important to you and deeply desired. Often changes are more likely to stick when the desire comes from within rather than directed by someone else. If you've ever tried to make a change, what was that like for you? In this chapter, we'll discuss how you can care for your diabetes *your way*. You can personalize your diabetes care by identifying changes *you* want to make. You'll have the opportunity to think critically about what's important to you (your values) and evaluate whether your current actions are lining up with these values. We'll also discuss the science behind behavior change and how our hard-wired thoughts and actions make change hard (but not impossible!). Fortunately, we can rewire and create new automatic thoughts and actions through some strategies that we'll discuss. In addition, we'll examine what gets in the way and how you can combat unconstructive thought patterns—such as all-or-nothing thinking—that keep you stuck.

Diabetes is a complex condition that affects individuals differently. This chapter will help you recognize your unique needs and build strategies for your own definition of success. The goal here is to make what's known about diabetes from advances in medicine and science match the realities of your personal needs and capabilities. Trying to do too much can leave you at risk for burnout—a state of exhaustion stemming from constantly feeling swamped. Are you ready to do diabetes care, your way?

Values Assessment: Living and Doing with Purpose

A value is a personal action or quality that you find important and meaningful. Values aren't internal states of mind or goals. For example, "feeling happy" isn't a value, but it might be a goal or desired internal state. Values are enduring, meaning you don't complete them and check them off a list. For example, if health is one of your values, you'll never finish doing things in the service of your health—it'll be an ongoing effort. Many values that we hold require ongoing attention, but being aligned with what's of most importance to you will feel worth the effort.

In chapter 3, you were invited to identify your top four values. What did you identify? How do the values you named relate to your diabetes care?

There's a well-known values metaphor about a classroom professor, though the original source is unknown. It goes as follows: A professor stands before his classroom with a large empty jar that he proceeds to fill with ping pong balls. Then he addresses his students and asks them if they think his jar is full. They all agree that it's full. Then he picks up a bag of small rocks and pours the rocks into the jar. The rocks fill in the spaces between the ping pong balls. He asks the class a second time if his jar is full, and again, they agree that it is. Next, the professor takes a bag of sand and pours it into the jar. The sand fills in the space between the ping pong balls and the rocks. For a third time, he asks his students if the jar is full, and they say it is. Finally, the professor produces two drinks and pours them into the jar, filling in any remaining spaces.

I invite you to consider how this metaphor applies to your life. The ping pong balls represent the things in your life that are of most value and are irreplaceable, such as your family, friends, and health. You must address them first. If you tried to fit ping pong balls into a jar full of sand, they wouldn't fit. Next, consider the little rocks. The rocks represent things of importance, but lesser importance than the ping pong balls. The rocks are replaceable things like your job and your car. The sand represents the small stuff, like having a tidy house or responding to every email. Some amount of the small stuff is inevitable, but if you spend too much of your time on things of little importance or value to you, you won't have time for the big things that really matter (Stoddard and Afari 2014). Lastly, the two drinks, as the story goes, is to show that no matter how full your life may seem, there's always room for a drink with a friend!

REFLECTION

Take a moment to consider your level of life balance. Many of the things at the sand level need to be done, but are you doing so at the expense of the ping pong balls?

Jim, an attorney, came to see me at the recommendation of his endocrinologist. His blood glucose and HbA1c were elevated to the prediabetes range, and he had a strong family history of diabetes. He was working eighty-plus-hour weeks, living off of coffee and take-out, barely sleeping, and almost never seeing his wife and two young children. He was exhausted and his wife was fed up. When we did a values assessment, it was clear to him that he was living out of alignment with his values. Rather than prioritizing his family, physical and mental health, friendships, and hobbies, he was making work his only focus. He decided to slowly make some shifts by setting some work boundaries, so that he could fill his jar with his ping pong balls first and the rocks and sand second and third. At our follow-up session two weeks later, he shared that he has made it a point to be home for family dinner each night, even if he still had to work a little more after the kids went to bed. He also gave himself a bedtime because he realized there will always be more work to do tomorrow; it might as well not come at the expense of his well-being.

The Stages of Change

Sometimes in my work with clients, I'll share with them that what I'm hearing from them reflects a particular stage of readiness to change. This can aid in our work together so that we are on the same page about any interest in changing a particular behavior. It would be unhelpful if I were to suggest actions to a client who was uninterested in making a particular change! Psychologists and researchers James Prochaska and Carlo DiClemente developed the transtheoretical model (also known as the "stages of change") in the late 1970s after observing individuals working on smoking cessation. They observed that individuals often move through five distinct stages to make a behavior change: precontemplation, contemplation, preparation, action, and maintenance (Prochaska and DiClemente 1985).

If you are in *precontemplation*, you have no intention of making a particular change in the foreseeable future; you may not even realize that there is something to change. In the *contemplation* stage, you recognize the need to make a change and are intending to change a behavior in the near future. In *preparation*, you are ready to take action toward a behavior change. If you've recently changed a behavior and intend to continue with it, then you are in the *action* stage. Finally, when a change has been sustained for a while (more than six months), you are in the *maintenance* stage of change.

This isn't necessarily a linear process. Take my client Rudy as an example. Rudy had maintained the addition of a twenty-minute walk after lunch on workdays for nearly a year when he went on a ten-day vacation to Mexico. While in Mexico, his routine was completely different, and he got out of the habit of doing his post-lunch walk. Once he returned to the office, he felt bogged down by catch-up work and skipped his lunch break altogether. When he realized that his blood sugar and stress levels were impacted by his new work-through-lunch routine, he again started making plans toward a change, moving back to the preparation stage once again.

REFLECTION

Think about a diabetes-related topic or health behavior. Can you assess where you are in your stage of change?

Combat Cognitive Distortions

Cognitive distortions are unhelpful, irrational thought patterns that can keep us feeling stuck and contribute to poor mental health. I don't think I've ever met someone who hasn't gotten stuck in these mental traps. Below, I've listed some common cognitive distortions I hear from my clients with diabetes, and some alternative thought statements:

- **Black-and-white (all-or-nothing, binary) thinking:** *I've already eaten too much, so I might as well just finish the plate.*

  Alternative: *I'm very full now, so I will leave the rest on my plate and eat it as leftovers tomorrow.*

- **Jumping to conclusions (mind reading):** *Everyone here is looking at me and judging my body size.*

  Alternative: *I'm having the thought that others are judging me, but in reality, I have no idea what others are thinking; and if they are judging me, that's their problem, not mine.*

- **Personalization:** *It's all my fault that I have this condition.*

  Alternative: *Diabetes is a complex condition that can develop due to a host of different predisposing factors out of my control.*

- **Fortune-telling:** *I just know my HbA1c will be too high, because it* always *is.*

Alternative: *I'll wait and see how my lab results look this time without making predictions.*

- **Catastrophizing:** *I keep forgetting to take my meds. I must be developing dementia!*

  Alternative: *Forgetfulness is common and doesn't necessarily mean dementia. However, it may be helpful to set up some reminders for myself in the future.*

- **"Should" statements:** *I really should be eating more vegetables.*

  Alternative: *It's been a while since I've had some good vegetables. Broccoli is nutritious and tasty when seasoned well and roasted with olive oil. I think I'll make some this weekend.*

- **Discounting the positive:** *I went for a walk today, but it was only ten minutes and that's not nearly long enough.*

  Alternative: *It was nice to get away from my desk to take a walk outside today. Even if it was shorter than I'd have liked, I know that even 10 minutes of walking has physical and psychological benefits.*

- **Overgeneralization:** *I'll never get my diabetes under control.*

  Alternative: *Diabetes management is hard work. I'll get my blood sugar in range with some new ideas from my team.*

Oftentimes, these cognitive distortions slip into our thoughts and take over before we've even noticed. To counter these unhelpful thoughts, see if you can notice they're happening before spiraling further into negative thought territory. One method I often invite my own clients to try is called *cognitive defusion,* which is a strategy that comes from ACT, a therapeutic approach briefly described in chapter 3. In this approach, the idea isn't to stop the thought from happening—which is nearly impossible to do, since thoughts are automatic—but to defuse, or filter, the unhelpful thoughts and not attach to them. There have been many metaphors developed to better envision this process, but one of my favorites is known as the "sushi train."

To visualize this metaphor, imagine that you are at a sushi restaurant in which sushi chefs prepare pieces of sushi and then place them on a conveyor belt that rotates in front of the restaurant patrons. As a patron, you pick up the sushi that looks appetizing to you and you leave the pieces that don't. Now, imagine that your thoughts are on this conveyor belt: some thoughts positive and helpful, some neutral, and others unhelpful and negative. When you pick up only the helpful and neutral thoughts, you are effectively defusing the negative thoughts by leaving them behind. Now, this probably sounds simple, but it certainly takes some practice and awareness. See if you can treat your brain and its thoughts like a sushi train today, filtering out the unhelpful thoughts and leaving the helpful ones. The more you practice this, the more automatic it will become to treat your thoughts in this way.

Understanding Behavior Change

Change takes effort, and it's not just about willpower. I often witness clients feeling upset with themselves because they haven't made a change they wanted to make. But just saying we want to do something isn't an automatic path to doing it. Renowned psychiatrist Daniel Siegel describes the focused attention that allows us to see the internal working of our minds as *mindsight* in his book by the same name. One concept that Siegel discusses in *Mindsight: The New Science of Personal Transformation* (2010) is neuroplasticity. Neuroplasticity is the ability your brain has to change and reorganize neural (nerve) pathways in response to stimuli and experiences. This is often described with the phrase "cells that fire together, wire together," which was coined by the late influential Canadian neuropsychologist Donald Hebb.

Let's look at a practical example of this concept of neuroplasticity. My client Gloria had developed many negative messages about food while growing up, and as a result, she avoided eating certain foods. However, sometimes her husband would buy something from her "avoid list" and she'd find herself breaking her own rules. When Gloria broke her food rules, she'd treat it like a "last supper," telling herself that she'd eat the food for the very last time. This created a feeling of scarcity, resulting in her eating to the point of feeling unwell and a corresponding spike in her blood sugar. Gloria had become used to this all-or-nothing behavior with her "avoid list" of foods.

Through our work together, Gloria began to understand and appreciate the principles of intuitive eating and was able to see that her mindset was limiting her ability to make peace with food and eat with attunement. But it wasn't enough to simply understand this on an intellectual level. To change the wiring of Gloria's brain and her automatic thoughts and behaviors around certain foods, she needed to *experience* eating these foods in new, peaceful ways.

To do this, we decided on some food exposures we'd do in our upcoming sessions together. We did several exposures together, using Gloria's most emotionally charged and shame-inducing foods. Gloria also practiced continuing to eat these foods outside of our sessions in planned experiences. After several months of practicing with one particular food, Gloria shared with me that eating it no longer led her to feel those negative emotions of the past. She said that now, when she ate the food, she was able to connect with the new experience she'd created through our exposure work. Her brain and nervous system's automatic response had changed through her new experiences as she unlearned old patterns and created new ones that built new neural pathways.

REFLECTION

Are there any thoughts or behaviors that you feel stuck around? How might you be able to bring attention and new experiences to these unwanted patterns?

Avoiding Burnout

Have you ever felt angry or frustrated about having diabetes? Maybe you've felt unmotivated to check blood sugars or keep up with your diabetes-related appointments. Perhaps at times you've felt like your efforts at self-care weren't making a difference or weren't seen as good enough.

Managing diabetes can be a lot to bear. The feelings I described above are common in people who are experiencing diabetes distress and burnout. If you have felt or currently feel this way, you aren't alone. Diabetes distress (burnout) affects one in four people with T1DM and one in five people with T2DM that use insulin. People with T2DM that aren't on insulin also experience this distress, but at a slightly lower rate of one in ten (Dennick et al. 2015).

If you've ever experienced a high level of distress related to your diabetes, what was that like? How are your self-care practices impacted when you're experiencing distress? Many people with diabetes who are experiencing high levels of distress describe disengagement from self-care tasks that were once automatic, such as taking meds or checking blood glucose. In addition, nutrition is often reported to suffer. When basic self-care behaviors slip up, sometimes eating behaviors take a turn toward unhelpful, with reports of binging or using food to cope. If you can relate, I invite you to explore intuitive eating principle seven with me: "cope with your emotions with kindness."

Cope with Your Emotions with Kindness

As described by *Intuitive Eating* authors Tribole and Resch, there are three paths to learn to cope with feelings without using food: 1) self-care, nurturance, and compassion; 2) learning to sit with emotions, and 3) helpful distraction (2020). Self-care and compassion are topics that were covered in chapter 3. As a quick recap, to be able to fully engage in care tasks, some fundamental needs must be met, such as getting enough sleep and rest, as well as cultivating pleasure, intellectual and creative stimulation, comfort, warmth, and the freedom to express feelings. Nurturance goes beyond self-care by doing extra for yourself—seeking out pleasurable experiences. Maybe this means seeking physical connection, reading a great book, making a point to watch the sunset, or taking a long, relaxing bath. Self-compassion involves treating yourself kindly and using curiosity rather than judgment when things don't go as intended. Take a second to evaluate your situation. Are you getting your basic human needs met? Are you doing things for enjoyment? Are you taking it easy on yourself when things don't go as planned? If you answered no to any of those questions, is there a small change you could make today, such as getting in bed ten minutes earlier than usual, cuddling with a loved one or pet for a few minutes, or giving yourself a kind response if your blood sugar check isn't in range?

Sitting with emotions takes practice. First, when you're having a strong emotion, can you pause to identify where in the body you feel it? You'll likely remember that the ability to identify felt senses within your body is known as interoceptive awareness. In chapter 2, we discussed interoceptive awareness as it relates to our ability to sense hunger, fullness, and satiety cues. Researchers have also studied this concept in relation to other felt senses, such as emotions. In 2018, a group of researchers out of Finland published a paper describing how they were able to map subjective feelings using topographical heat maps. These maps showed the human body with varying pixel intensities highlighting where emotions are felt in the body (Nummenmaa et al. 2018). I think the important message this study communicates is that emotions are felt in far-reaching parts of the body, not simply the head. What you might think of as a feeling or emotion limited to your mind is oftentimes felt in other areas of the body too. This could influence what you seek to satisfy bodily needs. For example, on the body feeling maps from the journal article, guilt, shame, and stress light up the brain and the entire torso. For some, this might mean seeking food despite not actually feeling hungry to satisfy the intense feeling in the abdomen. For others, it may be a desire to check out mentally and abandon usual care tasks, because of the intensity of the feeling in the head. Perhaps you have an automatic behavior that you jump to when you're feeling a particular emotion. Here's an optional experiment: the next time the urge to mentally check out or to eat in the absence of hunger comes, can you pause to first identify what you're feeling? Once you've recognized the feeling, you'll be better able to identify what you need.

For my client Cindy, she noticed that when she was feeling stressed, she'd automatically reach for something in her snack drawer at work. She said, "I'm definitely not hungry, I'm just nervous munching!" She decided she wanted to interrupt this automatic behavior by moving the snacks to a new location in her office. This way, when she didn't find snacks in the drawer, it would remind her to check in with her body and ask: *What am I feeling and what do I need?* At our follow-up session, she was excited to tell me that she'd done the experiment and it turned out that she just needed a break from her computer when she was reaching for her snack drawer. Taking the long route to the bathroom or a quick step outside did the trick, since she wasn't actually hungry in the first place. One thing that was also key here: Cindy knew she had full permission to eat a snack from the drawer if she ultimately decided that was what she needed. In Cindy's experience, she was treating her emotions with food when what she really needed was a break.

For some, distraction can be a helpful tool to use when identifying feelings and sitting with emotions is too much. While chronic avoidance of feelings often backfires, a temporary break from your feelings may be just what you need. It may be helpful to use distractions when you've had a hard day and really just want to get your mind off things or when you're feeling pained by a situation that's too fresh to process. My client Ruth actually put together a box of helpful distractions she could turn to when the time arose. As a middle school teacher, she often felt completely drained at the end of the day and sometimes just needed some distraction. Her box included fun coloring books and pencils, crafting supplies, fidget devices, sensory items like putty and crunchy paper, her favorite book of poetry, and some notes she wrote to herself. She appreciated having these items ready so that she didn't have to think of ideas when she was already deep in her feelings.

Personalizing Gentle Nutrition

Back in chapter 4, we covered the topic of gentle nutrition—making food choices that honor your health and taste buds while making you feel good. How and why you make food selections is an important aspect of doing diabetes care, your way. What guides you to make the food selections you do? In my experience working with clients, the most common factors cited for food choice selection included food accessibility, cost, convenience, culture, sensory factors, and health. Culture and sensory factors were covered back in chapter 3. Let's discuss some of the other factors below.

Accessibility and Cost

Do you have adequate access to the amount of food you need at all times? Food costs have been increasing, so if you're finding that more of your income is going to food costs, you're not alone. According to the consumer price index (CPI) for food, in 2022 food prices increased by nearly 10 percent, which was a faster rate of increase than any year since 1979. World events, such as avian influenza, affected egg and poultry prices. Additionally, conflicts in areas of the world that we depend on for certain imports also impacted these price escalations. However, all food price categories increased by more than 5 percent, outpacing historical averages for food price increases (USDA 2024). By the time you read this book, there may be new developments in the CPI. Regardless, here are a few tips that may help you in saving money at the grocery store.

First off, vegetarian proteins tend to be more cost effective than animal-based proteins. This doesn't mean you need to become a vegetarian! However, perhaps a meatless meal or two each week or adding veggie proteins to stretch meat dishes could help reduce costs. Dried beans, purchased in bulk, are an extremely nutrient-dense and cost-effective way to get protein. If you have a pressure cooker, you can cook beans without soaking them in about thirty minutes. Otherwise, they typically require an overnight soak and a slow simmer on the stove. If you want to try using beans to stretch a meat-based dish, you could add black beans to ground meat on taco night or some kidney beans to your turkey chili to get both a fiber boost and feed more mouths. In addition to beans, canned fish and ground turkey can serve as great additions to budget-conscious menus.

Like beans, grains are also often less expensive per ounce when purchased in bulk. Most grocery stores will list the price per ounce on the price tag so that you can compare products. Rice, oats, ground corn, and flour are some good, versatile grain options to keep on hand.

For fruits and vegetables, frozen is nearly always a cost-saving and nutrient-rich option. It's also a great way to continue enjoying fruits and veggies that are out of season. Frozen produce is picked at peak ripeness and frozen immediately, so it's usually more flavorful and may contain more micronutrients than the fresh versions, which often travel hundreds or thousands of miles before arriving at your local grocery store.

In terms of fresh produce, in-season options are going to be less expensive. For fruit, in general this means citrus in the winter, berries in the spring, stone fruits in the summer, apples and pears in the fall. Bananas tend to be available year-round and while prices vary by region and store, they generally cost less than thirty cents per banana. Also, canned tomatoes are a great addition to many dishes and are more cost effective than fresh varieties. They are harvested in season at peak ripeness and flavor, so canned tomatoes taste great and are a rich source of lycopene, a phytochemical with health benefits.

For fats, vegetable oil will be less expensive than olive oil, but the two have different culinary and nutritional purposes. If you can have both, I recommend a vegetable oil for high heat cooking and an olive oil for salad dressings, some baking, and medium heat cooking. For dairy, which is also an excellent protein source, you'll find that bulk purchases also offer some cost savings per ounce. Of course, dairy spoils much more rapidly than beans and grains, so you'll want to take into consideration if you'll be able to use a larger container before the expiration date. Pre-grated cheese or any type of food sold that had some labor or prep involved will also be more expensive per ounce. Purchasing a block of cheese, while requiring some additional effort, does save a bit of money.

In addition to the tips above, many product manufacturers have coupons on their websites. There are also grocery store apps that allow you to click e-coupons for use at checkout. Or, sign up for a rewards card (generally free) at your local grocery store to get additional discounts simply by swiping a card or entering your phone number. One of my favorite websites for budget-friendly recipe ideas is budgetbytes.com. This isn't a "diabetes recipe site," but keep in mind that people with diabetes don't need special foods and recipes. You can use your own knowledge of how your body responds to certain foods and amounts of foods to steer you toward certain recipes, but nothing is off-limits.

Convenience

A great meal can come together many different ways. It could be from scratch, partially from scratch, assembled from various ready-made ingredients, or fully prepped. None is better than the other. The best meal to land on your table is the one that works for you. Here are some ideas of how you might make these meal options work for you:

- **From-scratch cooking:** Cooking a meal from scratch could take anywhere from twenty minutes to multiple hours. It could be as simple as BBQ chicken with corn on the cob and a salad or as elaborate as homemade matzo ball soup. The sky's the limit here, but your time may dictate how elaborate your prep can be. Here are some great ideas for from-scratch cooking that have the added benefit of relative simplicity and fewer dirty dishes:

  - *Sheet-pan meals:* These are meals that can be 100 percent from scratch, but are such time- and clean-up savers because all ingredients get tossed onto one sheet pan and popped into the oven.

  - *One-pot meals:* Meals that cook all in one pot are similar in convenience to the sheet pan meals. There are many popular soups, pastas, curries, chilis, and rice dishes that can be made all in one pot.

BUDGET-FRIENDLY FOOD STAPLES

Proteins: dried beans, lentils, soy (tofu, edamame), peanut butter, eggs, canned fish (tuna, salmon, sardines), ground turkey

Produce: frozen fruits and veggies, canned tomatoes, fresh bananas, in-season fresh produce

Grains, starches: oats, rice, corn, pasta, potatoes, flour, bread

Fats: vegetable oil, extra virgin olive oil, butter, nuts and seeds, coconut milk

Dairy: milk, yogurt (large tub, plain), cheese (block), cottage cheese

Budget-Friendly Meal Ideas

Rice and beans topped with tomatoes, grated cheese, and a spoonful of sour cream

Oatmeal bake (oats baked with milk, frozen berries, egg, cinnamon) topped with a dollop of yogurt

Tofu and veggie (frozen broccoli and cauliflower) stir-fry (in vegetable oil) served with rice

Veggie egg scramble with cheese served alongside toast with butter

Lentil curry made with coconut milk, potatoes, frozen veggies

Tuna sandwich on whole-grain bread with a side of edamame

Pasta with a sauce made from seasoned canned tomatoes and ground turkey

- **Partially from scratch:** Assembling a meal that includes some ready-made items to create the meal is a real time-saver. This may mean using a rotisserie chicken from the store to make chicken enchiladas or jarred marinara sauce and boxed pasta to make spaghetti and meatballs.

- **Assembled from ready-made ingredients:** For further time saving, you can purchase prepped ingredients such as frozen microwaveable rice that's ready in 3 minutes, pre-chopped veggies, salad kits, pre-cooked meats, etc. For a quick, at-home burrito bowl, you could throw microwaved rice, canned beans, ready-made salsa, chopped romaine, shredded cheese, and a wedge of avocado together in less than 5 to 10 minutes.

- **Fully prepped:** I always suggest having several frozen items on hand for those days when you just need something fast or you're behind on getting fresh groceries. Some great options from the freezer section include burritos, pizzas, noodle dishes, fruits, veggies, chicken nuggets, meatballs, and more. You could quickly build a meal by adding a salad or some sauteed frozen veggies to a burrito or tossing in some frozen broccoli to a noodle dish as it's warming up.

Nutrition and Health

There are many ways to support your health through nutrition. With my clients, we focus on what to *add* rather than taking any food away. As we've discussed, restricting food contributes to the diet mentality, which will move you further away from intuitive eating. See if some of the following ideas might support any of your health-related concerns.

- Adding foods that slow down digestion, such as fat, protein, and fiber, to meals and snacks can help to slow the rise of blood glucose and keep you feeling satisfied for longer.

- .Resistant starches are starches that escape digestion. They are created when starchy foods, such as rice, pasta, bread, oatmeal, quinoa, potatoes, etc. are cooked and then chilled. This is known as starch retrogradation and may help improve your glycemic response to some foods. Research shows that fewer grams of carbohydrate are absorbed from the reheated starch. Food safety tip: be sure to keep foods out of the temperature danger zone of 40 degrees to 140 degrees Fahrenheit to avoid bacterial growth that can make you sick. That means refrigerate or freeze warm foods right away and then reheat to over 165 degrees Fahrenheit or steaming.

- If your cholesterol is high, adding more soluble fiber to your intake may help to lower it. Soluble fiber binds to cholesterol and allows it to be removed along with stool. It can be found in many plant foods, but is especially abundant in oats, legumes, oranges, Brussels sprouts, flaxseeds, psyllium husk, and avocado.

I met with Paul at the recommendation of his endocrinologist. Paul had a number of medical complications, one of which was diabetes. His HbA1c was sky-high and he was suffering from extreme fatigue and cognitive impairment as a result. When I met with Paul, he was not shy about telling me that he wasn't interested in "healthy eating." I told him that was fine and offered up a few ideas of things we could talk about. Through our conversation, I came to learn that he was not injecting any of his prescribed insulin because he had the idea that if he was eating "unhealthy," there was no point in taking his medication. He was experiencing a very dangerous all-or-nothing thought pattern. Once he understood that I wasn't going to tell him to stop eating his favorite foods, he became receptive to the idea of using his medication. He needed to do his diabetes care *his way*. When diabetes classes and doctors harped on the dos and don'ts of diabetes care, he shut down and decided to throw in the towel. But, with time, he was able to find his way of being intuitive with his food intake and his diabetes management. In the course of our work together, Paul moved from precontemplation to action.

REFLECTION

Think of an aspect of your diabetes self-care that you'd like to improve upon (self-monitoring, medication taking, eating, etc). What would you like to improve? What stage of change are you in when it comes to making this improvement?

Moving Forward

I hope you've gathered some ideas for doing diabetes care—your way. This chapter presented you with an opportunity to assess your values alignment, your interest in making a change, how to spot cognitive distortions, handling emotions, and a personalized approach to gentle nutrition. Next, we'll address the challenging topic of body image in chapter 8, "Navigating Body Image."

Navigating Body Image

The way you feel toward your body is known as your body image. Negative body image is a systemic, cultural issue—the result of living in a body-obsessed culture. A positive body image appreciates, accepts, and respects the unique beauty and function of your body even when it doesn't meet idealized images. It's feeling comfortable and confident in your body and emphasizing its assets rather than any imperfections (Wood-Barcalow, Tylka, and Augustus-Horvath 2010). Western societies are constantly promoting the "thin ideal," which leads many people to feel negatively about their bodies. When thinness also started becoming (incorrectly) associated with health, even more people were left striving to meet impossible body standards. I have many clients who tell me that love is too strong a word for them to associate with their bodies. You don't need to *love* your body, but can you respect it, care for it, stop fighting it, and maybe even accept it as is? This may feel like a radical idea to you, especially if you've been waging war with your body for some time. Tara Brach, a well-known psychotherapist and meditation teacher, describes *radical acceptance* as the willingness to experience ourselves and our life as it is (Brach 2003). This chapter will include an exploration of body image and a discussion of steps you may take to improve your relationship with your body by applying the key features of the intuitive eating principle, "respect your body."

Intuitive Eating Principle 8: Respect Your Body

Accept your genetic blueprint. Just as a person with a shoe size of eight would not expect to realistically squeeze into a size six, it is equally futile (and uncomfortable) to have the same expectation about body size. But mostly, respect your body so you can feel better about who you are. It's hard to reject the diet mentality if you are unrealistic and critical about your body size and shape. All bodies deserve dignity. (Tribole and Resch 2020)

You can show respect to your body by making it comfortable and by responding to its basic needs. Let's do a quick assessment to see how you're doing with body respect.

- Do you use body assessment tools, such as a scale?

- Are you wearing poorly fitting clothes?

- Are you using mirrors or measuring devices to scrutinize your body?

- Do you compare your body to others?

- Do you put your body down (out loud and/or in your thoughts)?

- Do you make adjustments to your intake based on how you feel about your body or what the scale says?

- Are you delaying or avoiding family photos, activities, celebrations, vacations, or clothing purchases because of your relationship with your body?

If you answered "yes" to any of the questions above, then we have some work to do toward increasing your level of body kindness. Many of the clients I've worked with over the years have also struggled with poor body image. For example, Kaitlyn had gotten into the habit of stepping on her bathroom scale first thing each morning from a young age. However, she was fed up with her morning mood being based on the number reflected back each day. When she'd finally had enough, she brought her scale into my office and said goodbye. All over the scale, she'd written parting messages, such as "my day won't be impacted by you," "I'm more than a number," and "I don't need you to start my day." In our subsequent counseling sessions, she described how free she felt without the scale exerting power over her. She was only truly able to begin listening to her body when she stopped receiving repeated input from her scale.

REFLECTION

What items or practices are currently exerting control over how you feel about your body? What can you do to make a change? Can you remove body assessment tools, such as scales? Do you need to delete tracking apps or cancel subscriptions? Maybe you need to alter who you follow on social media or what type of media you consume? If your clothes aren't fitting you comfortably or making you feel good, are you willing to address this?

"But My Clothes Don't Fit!"

For many clients I've worked with, a defining reason that they feel they must try to lose weight is that their clothes no longer fit. I can understand the frustration this brings. However, it still doesn't make the pursuit of weight loss safe or effective. Here, I'll propose a different path that addresses the present issue, which is the need for clothes that fit right *now*. Clothes are meant to fit *your body*, not the other way around.

If you've been telling yourself that your body needs to change to fit into a certain size, or into an old pair of jeans, what do you need to let go of that? The reality is that bodies change over time and it's unrealistic to expect our bodies to fit into clothes we wore many years ago. In addition, clothing brand sizing is anything but uniform! A size sixteen in one brand may be more like a size twelve in another. Let's aim to find clothing that fits well, makes you feel good, and is in line with your style preferences—without focusing on what the tag says.

For many, it feels unnerving to try and find something to wear in a closet full of clothes that won't fit today's body. Thus, the first order of business is a closet cleanout. Below, I've outlined some steps you may find helpful in initiating a closet cleanout when you're ready.

1. Pick one section or type of item to start with, such as pants. Sort through the pants you like and wear now and those that you don't wear and/or know aren't a fit for your body today.

2. Then, either: a) Store them in a labeled bin if you're not ready to get rid of them completely. At least they are out of the closet. Attach a note to the bin with the date. After six months or so, if you still haven't thought about or needed those clothes, maybe it's time to consider letting them go. b) Donate the clothes. Some companies will even come and pick your donations up from your doorstep. c) Use a resale site or consignment store to sell the clothes. If you do this, you can then earn some money to fund your new clothing purchases.

3. Repeat with other sections or types of clothing until your closet only holds clothes that fit you today. It's okay if you're left with a rather bare closet. We'll discuss finding new items below.

Next, it's time to start looking for replacement items. You'll be looking for clothes that make you feel good, are comfortable, and fit your here-and-now body. This doesn't have to break the bank. Many people find true gems at thrift and consignment stores or online at sites like Poshmark, Vinted, or ThredUp.

If you choose to purchase new clothes, you may consider whether you'd prefer to shop in person or online. For in-person shopping, consider going at a less crowded time of day, such as right when the store opens or on a weekday, if possible. Some stores, such as Nordstrom, have personal stylists who will assist you in finding what you need for no additional fee and no obligation to buy. My client Paula used this service when she needed several outfits for events leading up to her wedding and it really saved her time and the anguish of searching rack by rack for her style preference or size. Plus, she was able to find some great outfits that helped her to feel comfortable in her body.

If you're reluctant to shop in person, choose a store with online ordering and easy returns. Once you've found something you'd like to buy, check out the size chart and choose the size you think will fit. Then order the size (or two) above that as well. Once you receive your order, I'd suggest a no-look try-on in which you try on the item without looking at the size and waiting to look in the mirror. Before using a mirror, see how the clothing feels on your body. Move around in it. Sit down. Is it comfortable? Do you like the feel of the fabric? Wait until you've made these assessments to look in the mirror. At the mirror, aim to stay non-judgmental by noticing whether you like the color and the style. Can you see yourself wearing this out and feeling confident?

Kelly was a successful CEO and lifelong dieter. During one of our weekly sessions, she shared with me how much she truly despised all of her clothes and that even to big events, she'd wear her stretchy old yoga pants and throw a blazer on top. She didn't feel put together, and yet hadn't even considered buying new clothes because she kept telling herself that she must lose weight first. While she was working on eating intuitively, she also felt very negative about her body and truly wished for weight loss. What she eventually landed on is that she was open to trying a clothing subscription service, where she could share her preferences with a virtual stylist and receive a box of reasonably priced clothing options to try and either keep or send back. It felt helpful to Kelly that she didn't have to go to a store and deal with fitting rooms, salespeople, other customers, and a lack of size-inclusive options. She was thrilled with the items she received in her box—it was easy, affordable, and tailored to her style preferences and specific needs.

SIZE-INCLUSIVE BRANDS

Did you know that the majority of American women wear a size 16 or above (Christel and Dunn 2016)? Yet most brands stop at a size 14. That means shopping is a tough task for most. Fortunately, there are a few brands that have more inclusive size options. Here are a few, including the sizes they carry.

Universal Standard: up to 4XL or size 40

Lane Bryant: up to size 40

Madewell: up to 28W and 4X

Old Navy: up to size 30 or 4X online

Torrid: from size 10 to 30

Stitch Fix: up to 24W and 3X

Beyond Yoga: up to size 3X or 28

Athleta: up to 3X or 26

Girlfriend Collective: up to 6XL

Body Diversity

Even if we all ate the same type and amount of food and did the same amount of movement, we'd never have the same body size or weight. Yet, this is what many popular diets and influencers promise. They claim that if you just do as they say, you'll be on your way to matching a certain physique. What a lie! Diversity is what makes humans interesting and unique, whether it's skin color, height, body shape and size, or other appearance differences. Unfortunately, your own understanding and knowledge around body diversity won't stop the onslaught of thin-ideal messages and anti-fat sentiment around you. Below, I'll outline some common scenarios that may come up for you and provide some ideas for how you may decide to handle them.

- **Anti-fat bias and weight stigma in health care.** Health care is a human right, and yet many avoid checkups due to weight-stigmatizing care. You can use the resources provided in chapter 6 to see if you can find a weight-inclusive provider in your area. Or consider being an advocate for your needs. Refer back to the sample letter provided in the online tools at: https://www.IntuitiveEatingForDiabetes.com/resources for an example.

- **Concern trolling.** A *concern troll* offers criticism under the guise of concern. For example, "You really shouldn't eat that. I'm just concerned about your diabetes." Concern trolls need proper boundaries. Depending on your energy level, you might ignore the comment or let them know that no foods are off limits for you and your blood sugar is your business.

- **Body and diet talk.** It's uncomfortable when people around you are engaging in body bashing or diet talk when you're trying to be gentle with yourself. Maybe this happens when you're at lunch with friends or when you go home for the holidays. Whatever the circumstance, it'll feel good to be prepared to deal with the situation. You could opt to change the subject, set a boundary on conversation topics, or, if you're feeling up to it, provide some intuitive eating education to the person who's bringing up their latest diet.

Mourning the Fantasy Body

There are many challenges to having a body, especially if you've ever had a rupture in your relationship with your body. A rupture may occur if your body isn't meeting your expectations. Perhaps you've sustained an injury, or you live with a permanent disability that has affected the way you feel toward your body. Living with diabetes means living with a chronic medical condition; does this impact your feelings toward your body? Perhaps you feel negatively toward your appearance, attributes, abilities, disabilities, performance, or functionality. Maybe you used to feel great about your body, but that changed as you got older and experienced the various inevitabilities of aging. You aren't alone in your feelings.

Has your body ever let you down? For many, diabetes can feel like a big bodily letdown. Maybe you've asked yourself in frustration, "Why can't my body just function as it's supposed to?" From my experience working with clients on their intuitive eating journeys, one of the hardest parts centers around body acceptance. This is especially challenging in a culture that fancifully worships thinness as ideal for both beauty and health.

Diabetes and Body Image

How does having diabetes impact your body image? A handful of studies addressing body image and diabetes have been published to date. Polish researchers Kokoszka et al. (2022) found that when compared with the general population of Poland, people with diabetes have worse body image, which was observed to be significantly related to HbA1c levels and diabetes-related distress. Wirth et al. (2014) found that chronic dissatisfaction with one's body weight, regardless of BMI, was associated with an *increased* risk of T2DM.

With body appreciation comes a natural tendency to pay attention to internal bodily needs, such as eating according to hunger and fullness cues, a hallmark of intuitive eating (Avalos and Tylka 2006). In line with this, a systematic review found intuitive eating to be associated with less disordered eating and a more positive body image (Bruce and Ricciardelli 2016). Herzog Ramos et al. (2022) found that trusting hunger and satiety cues doubled the chances of body satisfaction in people with T2DM. Body satisfaction means accepting, respecting, and having a favorable opinion of one's own body, as well as rejecting unrealistic body ideals. On the flip side, negative thoughts and feelings about one's body are defined as body dissatisfaction, which is considered to be the most important global measure of stress related to the body (Quittkat et al. 2019). In sum, these studies found intuitive eating to be associated with improved body image, which may be associated with better diabetes markers.

Is your body image impacted by any diabetes devices you use as part of your self-management routine? Diabetes technology has advanced tremendously over the years and there are now more wearable devices available. Some of these are visible to others, which may make you feel a particular way. Many clients I've worked with have grappled with this. While visible tech on your body may make you feel like a standout among others, the more you hide it, the less the public will ultimately understand the unique differences among people in our world. If you find yourself hiding your condition, I challenge you to do some exposure work around allowing more of your diabetes management needs to be visible in public. Can you check your blood sugar with a glucometer at the table? Can you wear a sleeveless shirt that exposes your CGM sensor? Can you take diabetes oral meds while seated in a restaurant among friends? Can you give yourself insulin in plain sight at the next family gathering? In what way do you hide your diabetes? There's no shame in having diabetes. By hiding your self-management needs, are you communicating a lack of acceptance and a feeling of shame? Perhaps hiding less would foster a greater acceptance and more positive feelings toward your body.

Even with acceptance and a willingness to let your diabetes be more visible, you likely still feel frustrated with the need to poke and prod or change tubes or be connected to devices. Maybe you've developed self-management side effects, such as lipohypertrophy—a lump of fatty tissue under the skin caused by repeated injections in the same place—and feel embarrassed or angry about it. It's understandable to feel frustrated about these things. Can you grieve and offer self-compassion too?

Grieving the Thin Ideal

Are you familiar with Elisabeth Kübler-Ross's seminal book, *On Death and Dying* (2009)? In it, Kübler-Ross outlines five stages of grief related to one's own death or the death of a loved one: denial, anger, bargaining, depression, and acceptance. Since her original description of these stages, the model has been applied to many other reactions to significant change or upheaval, one of which is *grieving the thin ideal*. Jeanne Courtney (2008) wrote about size acceptance as a grieving process from the vantage point of her work as a psychotherapist. Inspired by her paper, counselor Meredith Noble (n.d.) wrote about this topic in a blog post titled "Body Acceptance Begins with Grieving the Thin Ideal." I have shared this piece countless times with clients over the years.

Here's how these stages of grief have shown up for my clients with regards to weight and may for you, too:

- **Denial:** In this stage, you might be thinking, *Of course I can lose weight; I've done it before!* You may think this despite your own lived experiences with weight cycling, wanting to believe it'll be different this time.

- **Anger:** It's very understandable to feel angry if you've been dieting and restricting for some time, only to discover that diets don't work and the weight cycling that ensues is especially harmful.

- **Bargaining:** If you find yourself stating, "I just want to lose some weight first and then work on intuitive eating," then you are in the bargaining stage.

- **Depression:** Perhaps you're feeling depressed about the time, money, and energy you spent focusing on weight loss to no avail. It's not your fault if you got caught up in diet culture or tried to follow the advice you were given by health professionals in your life who said that you had to lose weight to be healthy.

- **Acceptance:** When you've landed here, you've accepted the fact that striving for weight loss is harmful and you can take care of your diabetes without trying to shrink your body.

While you grieve, know that the process may not be linear. You may get to acceptance, only to be shuttled back into the denial phase again when a new fad that promises to be different gains popularity. When that happens, self-compassion is in order: *Of course I'm feeling tempted to jump on another "quick fix" because of the cultural obsession with weight, but I know what my body needs to function best.*

Exposure Work

If you, like most of us, have grown up seeing thinness praised and fatness vilified, then you likely have some anti-fat bias to work through. Everyone has biases, whether they want to or not. An experience that has stuck with me for decades is that of visiting the Simon Wiesenthal Center's Museum of Tolerance in Los Angeles, CA. At the entrance to one of the first exhibits are two doors. Patrons are to choose a door to go through: the door that says "biased" or the door that says "not biased." Most people try to go through the door labeled "not biased," but that door is locked. Thus, all museumgoers are shuttled through the door labeled "biased." There is a powerful lesson in this experience: everyone holds biases. It's up to us to see our biases and choose actions that align with our values rather than the bias we hold.

When it comes to body biases, powerful and mindset-shifting work can be done through exposure to diverse bodies. When our culture promotes conventionally attractive, thin, and able bodies, our brains get wired to think those bodies are best or "normal." Because of this, we may feel negative and judgmental of our own bodies that don't look like those we see promoted by the media.

Contact hypothesis states that under the right conditions, social contact between different groups can improve intergroup relations (Allport 1954). Alperin et al. (2014) applied the contact hypothesis to the field of weight bias and found that, consistent with the contact hypothesis, when participants in their study had positive contact with people in larger bodies, they had more positive attitudes toward them. However, negative contact with people in larger bodies led to even stronger anti-fat attitudes. It's no wonder that anti-fat sentiment is so rampant when you consider the body sizes of various cartoon villains and other negative tropes applied to larger-bodied people in the media (think Ursula, Uncle Phil, "Fat Amy," Homer

Simpson). A form of exposure therapy can be as simple as adding more contact with people across the size spectrum doing positive things and living joyous lives. This could be as simple as following certain accounts on social media. On Instagram, this includes accounts such as @iamchrissy king, @theunderbellyyoga, @curvyyoga, @v_solesmith, @yrfatfriend, @theshirarose, and @thebodypositive, to name just a few. On TV, this includes shows such as *Shrill* and *Dietland*, both based on books by the same names. The visual experience of seeing people in larger bodies who are embracing life rather than trying to shrink their bodies can be mindset-shifting.

Another type of exposure that's used to address negative body image is mirror exposure therapy (Griffen, Naumann, and Hildebrandt 2018). This involves viewing one's body in a mirror using specific guidance. It's a validated treatment for improving body image and satisfaction. One way of conducting mirror exposure is to look in the mirror and describe your reflection, starting from the top of your body, using descriptive but non-judgmental language. For example, if I were to do this, I might say: "I have straight, shoulder-length brown hair, parted to the side; thin, mildly arched eyebrows; brown almond-shaped eyes; an oval-shaped face with fair skin and some scattered freckles," and so forth. Notice that I gave neutral descriptions, not negative judgments. Do you want to give it a try? If you do, please stop your process if you notice negative language emerging. You can come back to it another day and see how far you get without judgments slipping in.

Navigating Body Changes with Diabetes

It's inevitable that your body will change over time. Beauty culture will have you believe that you can stop aging by investing in its products, treatments, and services. However, there's a limit to the effects of even the most expensive and invasive procedures. Body changes are par for the course, affected by medical conditions, medications, age, a return to adequate eating (from inadequate), and even improving blood sugars. Weight gain can occur when you get your blood sugars under better control because improved blood sugar means your body is able to utilize more nutrition from the food you eat.

I worked with twenty-six-year-old Ellie when she'd just finished law school and was engaged to be married. She'd had T1DM since childhood. Her dad had it too, and unfortunately passed down plenty of misinformation about the condition to his daughter. Ellie grew up in a household where thinness was praised. When Ellie's body changed from her childhood thin physique to her womanly curvy body, she felt criticized. Ellie also struggled with her mental health and black-and-white thinking so she often veered back and forth between restriction and binge eating. When she was restricting, she'd be meticulous with her diabetes care, but when binging, she'd feel so ashamed of her actions that she'd often omit insulin completely. Her diabetes was not under control, and she was in a shame spiral.

She reached out to me because she wanted to start taking care of her body and her diabetes. To do this, she needed to start giving her body the amount of insulin it needed. Ellie knew that her practice of withholding insulin was very dangerous and damaging, but she feared the weight gain that would come with better nourishment. With some grieving of the thin ideal, Ellie was slowly able to accept her nourished body more and more. She bought new clothes and got rid of her "sick clothes." She even purchased a new wedding dress when she realized that the dress she'd purchased a year prior was not going to work for her body now that she was fully caring for it. After the wedding, she sent me a few photos and said, "I'm looking at these images with new and kinder eyes."

REFLECTION

What's your body story? If you think of your body as a tree, what would lie under the soil and up in the leaves? In your companion journal, I invite you to diagram your own tree and roots. What is your relationship with your body like today (leaves) and what has shaped this relationship (roots)?

Moving Forward

This chapter has introduced you to various ways in which you might work to develop a better relationship with your body. It'll take time and continued practice to improve this relationship. Be patient with yourself. Offer yourself compassion while navigating this process. Consider the valuable qualities you possess, such as your intelligence, work ethic, kindness, generosity, humor, or other traits. Ultimately, shifting your focus to things beyond physical appearance will benefit you greatly. Don't let how you feel about your body prevent you from taking the vacation, getting in the photo, going to the class reunion, and doing all the things that add quality to your life. Perhaps you can practice radical acceptance of your body as it is; after all, it's the only one you get. You might need to revisit this chapter many times and that's okay; this process often isn't linear. In the next and final chapter, you'll hear from three people with diabetes who took the intuitive path and what it was like for them.

CHAPTER 9

Intuitive Eating with Diabetes in the Real World

Throughout this book, I've shared the experiences of various clients I've worked with via short case examples. In this final chapter, I'll introduce you more closely to three clients that worked with me one-on-one for a total of nearly five years between them. These individuals have been generous enough to share what it was like for them to re-learn how to be intuitive eaters while managing diabetes because they want you, the reader, to truly understand that it's possible for you too. You'll hear from Magnolia, who found intuitive eating around the time of her T2DM diagnosis; David, whose long dieting history led him to seek food freedom through an intuitive eating practice just before being diagnosed with T2DM; and finally you'll hear from Peyton, who's had T1DM since age nine. Each has identified intuitive eating as a savior from the dark place where mainstream diabetes recommendations and diet culture collide. As I beam the spotlight on these brave individuals with diabetes who took the intuitive eating path, you'll hear the anecdotes, stories, and wisdom that they've allowed me to share with you.

Magnolia

Magnolia was twenty-two years old when she was diagnosed with T2DM. It felt overwhelming and shame-inducing to receive this diagnosis. She'd already been dealing with an eating disorder that began in childhood. The diabetes medical community didn't feel like an option to her—there was too much fear-mongering. She knew the restrictive ways of traditional diabetes management just wouldn't work, especially given her own rocky history with food and body image. Fortunately, she had a therapist who'd recommended *Intuitive Eating* years prior. So instead of going to a diabetes class, she began learning about intuitive eating, which felt safer and more accessible. Magnolia reflects on this choice of using intuitive eating to manage her diabetes now, ten years later:

> I struggled intensely with shame and stigma about being diagnosed with diabetes when I was twenty-two due to experiences of weight-based abuse in childhood and societal messages. I was also at a point with my eating disorder where I recognized that my life had become unmanageable and felt continuing on the roller coaster of weight cycling, restriction, binging, and the like was unsustainable. It was a point of desperation for me because I was not able to manage it on my own. I did some research and began to understand that the typical weight loss prescription for diabetes was not available or doable for me, because my eating disorder was only going to get worse—and subsequently, my health as well.
>
> The way I feel when I look back on these experiences of diving into intuitive eating in the face of a new diabetes diagnosis is that I lost the fight but won the war. In my process following the intuitive eating steps I did initially gain some weight, which was difficult for me mentally at the time, but ten years later, I have better health at thirty-two than I did at twenty-two, long-term stability in my body, and my mind is peaceful instead of being consumed with thoughts of food. My mental bandwidth has expanded so much in these years because I'm able to focus on

other areas of my life, including healing and growing as a person in ways that were not available to me prior.

Food is still a little bit logistically complicated because of other reasons like budget, time, and family members with different preferences and needs, but there is no longer anguish or chaos involved with food in my life. And for that, I am so incredibly grateful. I genuinely don't think I would have made it to thirty-two without intuitive eating, because I was not able to cope with my life and my eating disorder at the same time. Life, and diabetes, are more manageable for me now because I chose to take a long-term view of my health instead of the short-term benefits that weight loss could provide, but subsequently worsen over time. I have successfully managed my diabetes for ten years while doing intuitive eating, and I plan to continue this way.

It's a bit emotional, this reflection, but I think it is the most meaningful thing I can say about my journey with diabetes and intuitive eating. *I think it saved my life.*

Magnolia isn't the first person to share that intuitive eating has saved their life. It's profound to know that kicking diet culture to the curb can unleash so much more potential for happiness, that a whole undiscovered world opens up! Eating disorders are, in fact, the deadliest of all mental illnesses, so it makes sense that finding food freedom and body peace is lifesaving (Smink, van Hoeken, and Hoek 2012).

This can be true whether you've had an eating disorder or not. In fact, this was demonstrated in a landmark study from the 1940s called the Minnesota Starvation Experiment. Subjects in this study spent the first three months of the study consuming a typical, nourishing diet before their caloric intake was subsequently cut by more than half. The researchers were surprised by the psychological effects observed during this semi-starvation period. The hunger the subjects endured led to obsessive behaviors around food: they'd dream, fantasize, and talk about food; they'd savor meals by eating slowly and cutting food up into little bites; and they were irritable, depressed, and apathetic (Baker and Keramidas 2013). Have you ever experienced anything similar from dieting or restricting your food intake? I wouldn't be surprised if you did—the level of caloric restriction in the Minnesota Starvation Experiment is actually similar to many weight-loss plans that dieters endure. This is why intuitive eating is lifesaving work! Food restriction leads to poor psychological and physical health. The peace and happiness that results from re-nourishment is life-altering.

Magnolia was wise enough to know that she couldn't endure more restriction and was fortunate enough to land on intuitive eating as a way out of diet culture and into a positive relationship with food. Today, she is enjoying life with her partner. Things aren't perfect, because they don't need to be, yet she is able to eat intuitively and her diabetes is managed. Magnolia's advice to you: be gentle with yourself.

David

David and I had already been working together regularly on intuitive eating for a couple years when he was diagnosed with diabetes and started on insulin. For him, restrictive eating and dieting had started in child-hood. Since he'd just spent over a year working to remove restrictions and add flexibility to his eating, he was understandably concerned. With a new diabetes diagnosis, he was now unsure whether he'd be able to continue eating intuitively and manage his blood sugar. All around him, he was hearing that with diabetes, there was a certain way to eat, and it was bring-ing back very unpleasant memories of his restrictive eating past.

Together, we worked through the messages he was getting from his endocrinology clinic and what he knew to be true for him as an intuitive eater. His nurse practitioner (NP) at the clinic was asking him to drasti-cally limit carbs in a way that felt unreasonable and reminded him way too much of being on a diet. David wanted to know how he could eat a more satisfying amount of carbs and keep his blood sugars in check. His NP had prescribed him a set insulin bolus to match the restricted carb amount she'd instructed him to eat, which was limiting him. What he really needed was a flexible insulin regimen using a carb-to-insulin ratio rather than the rigid set insulin and carb prescription he'd been given. With an insulin-to-carb ratio, he'd be able to be more intuitive with his carb intake. To use the ratio, he'd need to be able to add up the carb grams he consumed and then calculate his insulin dosage. For example, if his carb-to-insulin ratio was 1 to 10 and he ate a meal that contained 70 grams of carbohydrate, he'd know to inject 7 units of insulin. Then, if at the next meal, he only ate 40 grams of carbs, he'd inject 4 units. This would allow him the ability to eat flexibly, in line with intuitive eating.

David was excited about the potential to eat intuitively and adjust his insulin accordingly, so I connected with his NP to collaborate on this plan. Fortunately, she was receptive, and set us up with an insulin-to-carb ratio for David to use going forward. These ratios need to be personalized, as they'll vary based on one's insulin sensitivity. In general, one unit of rapid-acting insulin will cover 12–15 grams of carbohydrate, but this can range from 5 to over 30 grams. In addition, insulin sensitivity can vary based on time of day (e.g., it's common to be more insulin resistant in the morning), stress, and physical activity. If you're on insulin and don't use an insulin-to-carb ratio, but would like to, talk about this with your health care team.

David and I concluded our work together when he was at a point of confidence with his intuitive eating practice and ability to manage his blood sugar. When I reconnected with him for this book, what he really wanted to convey to you, reader, is this: "It's possible to manage diabetes using intuitive eating. You don't have to succumb to diet culture and classic diabetes management approaches." David emphasized that learning to manage diabetes is a marathon, not a sprint. He found that experimentation with food combinations was key to learning how his blood sugar would respond. In some ways, this felt like more work than just following the carb restrictive advice, but now that he's at a place where it feels intuitive, he knows it was worth the exploratory effort and will likely aid in preventing burnout.

In addition, David found it necessary to be an advocate for his needs at the doctor's office. He had to make it very clear that he wasn't going to take their weight-centric, restrictive approach. This wasn't always easy, especially because he wasn't able to find a supportive community for weight-inclusive diabetes outside of our sessions, but he stood his ground. Today, he is enjoying the freedom that intuitive eating has brought to his diabetes care.

Peyton

Peyton reached out to me for nutrition counseling during the fall of 2020 when the COVID-19 pandemic was still in full swing. We met via tele-health regularly for the next year until she moved out of state. When we concluded our work together, she shared this: "I have to say [learning to eat intuitively with diabetes] has changed my entire life. I eat with complete freedom now and my HbA1c has remained steady [in the 7's rather than up in the 11's]. There is a complete change in the way I see myself. You helped me do the impossible and I'm forever grateful."

When Peyton and I began working together, she was in a negative place with her eating and body image. She'd just graduated college and was engaged to be married; there were so many positive things happening in her life, yet she was really struggling with her diabetes and relationship with food. She'd picked up many rules around food, carbs, and diabetes in the time since she was diagnosed with T1DM at age nine. To her, there were only a certain amount of carbohydrate grams that were acceptable to eat with diabetes and she felt immense shame and embarrassment if she ate beyond that amount. Instead of giving herself the amount of insulin needed for the actual amount of carbs consumed, she'd bolus for the amount she *thought* she should've eaten. This led to a constant mismatch between insulin and carb intake, and thus high blood sugar levels after eating. The morality around carb intake for her, alongside a lot of all-or-nothing thinking, resulted in a recurrent binge/restrict pattern.

Peyton felt a lot of sadness about having diabetes. In some ways, she felt like her body had failed her. It felt embarrassing to wear medical devices or to have low blood sugar around others. In addition, she was feeling burnt out, between twelve years of diabetes, moving away from home, completing a rigorous college degree in three years, and a global pandemic.

We took our work together one step at a time. The first thing we addressed was giving insulin for the amount of carbs consumed. It was helpful for Peyton to think of her job of bolusing as simply doing what her pancreas would have been doing if it was still able to produce insulin. She found it useful to keep in mind that when others eat a bowl of pasta, their bodies just send out the insulin needed to match that carb load, which keeps blood sugars in range. She began to understand that it was up to her to act as her body's pancreas and there was no shame in eating more than a particular amount of carbs if that's what she needed. Our bodies aren't robots that need the same amount of food at each meal.

As Peyton began to get her blood sugar in better control, her body was getting the vital nutrition that it needed. This meant she noticed some body changes as well. Because she had a wedding coming up, she had some family shopping events planned. Peyton was able to set boundaries with family regarding body commentary and shared her preferences with the salespeople. In addition, she planned for a no-look try-on that would allow her to try clothes on and assess for comfort without attention to the size on the tag. As the big day was getting closer, we even developed a plan for looking at pictures with kind eyes. Peyton identified that she wanted to see love and happiness reflected back in her photos rather than feeling a need to scrutinize her body. She was able to stay connected to her values by engaging in cognitive defusion when unhelpful thoughts about her body surfaced. For example, instead of "my face looks too big in that photo," she was able to rephrase it as "*I'm having the thought that* my face looks big in that photo." This re-phrasing was able to remind her that this was an unhelpful thought (and judgment), not a fact.

Another aspect of our body image work involved exposure to different types of bodies. Like most Americans, Peyton felt very influenced by the thin ideal that is predominant in mainstream media. When our brains are constantly bombarded by messaging that promotes the idea that thin is better, it can be hard to see outside that viewpoint. Fortunately, there are a number of outlets that are helping to make real bodies more visible. Some examples include the previously mentioned TV show *Shrill*, the film *Your Fat Friend, the 4th Trimester Bodies Project,* various social media accounts, and children's books such as *Bodies Are Cool* by Tyler Feder, which features bodies that are large and small, disabled and able-bodied, and skin that is dark, light, or with vitiligo. Peyton opted to read a book I'd recommended, *The Body Is Not an Apology* by Sonya Renee Taylor, and found it to be very helpful in her body image journey.

After over a year of regular nutrition counseling sessions, Peyton and I were able to close our work together. She'd successfully learned how to apply intuitive eating principles to better manage her T1DM and she was feeling more at peace with food and her body. As part of our closing work, she created a list of the noticeable improvements she experienced when she ate regularly, which included: more energy, better able to be kind to herself and others, improved mental health, able to be productive with work, improved relationships, not constantly thinking about food, and superior blood sugar results. She plans to come back to this list whenever she needs a reminder that will keep her connected to her intuitive eating practice.

Moving Forward

I hope hearing from Magnolia, David, and Peyton has given you some hope and assurance that you, too, can use intuitive eating principles to guide your diabetes management. What can you take from each of their experiences that may feel applicable in your own life?

We've been on quite a journey together in these nine chapters, covering the nuts and bolts of diabetes, the four pillars of intuitive eating for diabetes management, and creating a personalized diet-free lifestyle. Please remember to be kind to yourself through this process—learning to eat intuitively is hard work, and even more challenging when there's a medical condition on board. I'd recommend revisiting chapters and concepts as needed. Intuitive eating is a practice, so just like anything in life, we have to keep practicing to perform in accordance with our goals. In this case, practice leads to improvement, but we're not aiming for perfection.

Acknowledgments

I'm extremely grateful to Ryan Buresh, Vicraj Gill, and the entire New Harbinger team for seeing my vision in this book and helping me to get it out into the world.

To my clients, past and present—thank you for your vulnerability and allowing me to be a guide on your journey. I have and continue to learn so much from you. Extra thanks go out to Magnolia, David, and Peyton for their immense generosity in sharing their lived experiences with intuitive eating and diabetes.

I'm indebted in gratitude toward Evelyn Tribole and Elyse Resch for not only writing the groundbreaking *Intuitive Eating* book back in 1995 and each of its subsequent editions, but for also being my mentors and teachers over the years. Thank you for entrusting me to apply the ten principles you created to diabetes care.

A special thanks to my long-time colleague and friend, Sumner Brooks, who read my book proposal while on vacation and provided lightning-speed feedback! I so appreciated your words of encouragement and check-ins along this journey.

To all of my weight-inclusive colleagues and researchers, thank you for doing the immensely important work you do. Special thanks to researchers Tracy L. Tylka, Rebecca L. Pearl, Catherine P. Cook-Cottone, and Erin D. Basinger, who graciously communicated with me via email during the book writing process.

I am tremendously thankful to my mom for instilling a fierce work ethic in me from a young age and for always being my cheerleader.

To my two amazing children, you inspire me every day and I love you more than you'll ever know.

Last but certainly not least, thank you to my dedicated husband, who always believes in my wild ideas and graciously read every single chapter draft I handed him and provided his honest feedback. You're my rock.

References

Abugoukh, T. M., A. Al Sharaby, A. O. Elshaikh, M. Joda, A. Madni, I. Ahmed, et al. 2022. "Does Vitamin D Have a Role in Diabetes?" *Cureus* 14(10): e30432.

Abushukur, Y., C. Cascardo, Y. Ibrahim, F. Teklehaimanot, and R. Knackstedt. 2022. "Improving Breast Surgery Outcomes Through Alternative Therapy: A Systematic Review." *Cureus* 14(3): e23443.

ADCES. "ADCES7 Self-Care Behaviors." Accessed August 24, 2023. https://www.adces.org/diabetes-education-dsmes/adces7-self-care-behaviors.

Adesoba, T. P., and C. C. Brown. 2023. "Trends in the Prevalence of Lean Diabetes Among US Adults, 2015–2020." *Diabetes Care* 46(4): 885–889.

Allport, G.W. 1954. *The Nature of Prejudice.* Cambridge, MA: Addison-Wesley.

Alperin, A., M. J. Hornsey, L. E. Hayward, P. C. Diedrichs, and F. K. Barlow. 2014. "Applying the Contact Hypothesis to Anti-Fat Attitudes: Contact with Overweight People Is Related to How We Interact with Our Bodies and Those of Others." *Social Science & Medicine* 123: 37–44.

Amazon. n.d. "Dietary Supplements." Accessed February 1, 2024. https://sellercentral.amazon.com/gp/help/external/55N3JF2WQS7RVNE.

American Diabetes Association. 2017. "Pharmacologic Approaches to Glycemic Treatment." *Diabetes Care* 40(Suppl 1): S64–S67.

———. 2023. "Classification and Diagnosis of Diabetes: *Standards of Care in Diabetes—2023.*" *Diabetes Care* 46(Suppl 1): S19–S40.

Ärnlöv, J., B. Zethelius, U. Risérus, S. Basu, C. Berne, B. Vessby, G. Alfthan, and J. Helmersson. 2009. "Serum and Dietary β-Carotene and α-Tocopherol and Incidence of Type 2 Diabetes Mellitus in a Community-Based Study of Swedish Men: Report from the Uppsala Longitudinal Study of Adult Men (ULSAM) Study." *Diabetologia* 52: 97–105.

Asbaghi, O., N. Fatemeh, R. K. Mahnaz, G. Ehsan, E. Elham, N. Behzad, A.-L. Damoon, and A. N. Amirmansour. 2020. "Effects of Chromium Supplementation on Glycemic Control in Patients with Type 2 Diabetes: A Systematic Review and Meta-Analysis of Randomized Controlled Trials." *Pharmacological Research* 161: 105098.

Avalos, L. C., and T. L. Tylka. 2006. "Exploring a Model of Intuitive Eating with College Women." *Journal of Counseling Psychology* 53(4): 486–497.

Bacon, L. 2010. *Health at Every Size: The Surprising Truth About Your Weight*, 2nd ed. Dallas, TX: BenBella Books.

Bacon, L., and L. Aphramor. 2011. "Weight Science: Evaluating the Evidence for a Paradigm Shift." *Nutrition Journal* 10: 9.

Baker, D., and N. Keramidas. 2013. "The Psychology of Hunger." *Monitor on Psychology* 44(9): 66.

Balducci, S., M. Sacchetti, J. Haxhi, G. Orlando, V. D'Errico, S. Fallucca, S. Menini, and G. Pugliese. 2014. "Physical Exercise as Therapy for Type 2 Diabetes Mellitus." *Diabetes/Metabolism Research and Reviews* 30(S1): 13–23.

Basinger, E. D., S. J. Cameron, and G. Allen. 2023. "Stigma, Self-Care, and Intuitive Eating in Black Americans with Type 2 Diabetes." *Journal of Racial and Ethnic Health Disparities*, August 25.

Bennett, B., and R. M. Puhl. 2023. "Diabetes Stigma and Weight Stigma Among Physicians Treating Type 2 Diabetes: Overlapping Patterns of Bias." *Diabetes Research and Clinical Practice* 202: 110827.

Berchtold, P., P. Bolli, U. Arbenz, and G. Keiser. 1969. "Disturbance of Intestinal Absorption Following Metformin Therapy (Observations on the Mode of Action of Biguanides." *Diabetologia* 5(6): 405–12.

Birch, L. L., S. L. Johnson, G. Andresen, J. C. Peters, and M. C. Schulte. 1991. "The Variability of Young Children's Energy Intake." *New England Journal of Medicine* 324(4): 232–235.

Bogusch, L. M., and W. H. O'Brien. 2019. "The Effects of Mindfulness-Based Interventions on Diabetes-Related Distress, Quality of Life, and Metabolic Control Among Persons with Diabetes: A Meta-Analytic Review." *Behavioral Medicine* 45(1): 19–29.

Brach, T. 2003. *Radical Acceptance: Embracing Your Life with the Heart of a Buddha.* New York: Bantam.

Britannica, T. Editors of Encyclopaedia. 2024. "Adolphe Quetelet." *Encyclopedia Britannica*, April 3. https://www.britannica.com/biography/Adolphe-Quetelet.

Brown, H. 2015. *Body of Truth: How Science, History, and Culture Drive Our Obsession with Weight—and What We Can Do About It.* Boston: Da Capo Lifelong.

Bruce, L. J., and L. A. Ricciardelli. 2016. "A Systematic Review of the Psychosocial Correlates of Intuitive Eating Among Adult Women." *Appetite* 96: 454–472.

Brush, M. 2021. "Amazon as Crystal Ball: Can Natural Brands and Retailers Use E-Commerce to Predict Trends?" *Nutrition Business Journal* 13–15.

Budiastutik, I., H. M. Subagio, M. I. Kartasurya, B. Widjanarko, A. Kartini, Soegiyanto, and S. Suhartono. 2022. "The Effect of Aloe Vera on Fasting Blood Glucose Levels in Pre-Diabetes and Type 2 Diabetes Mellitus: A Systematic Review and Meta-Analysis." *Journal of Pharmacy & Pharmacognosy Research* 10(4): 737–747.

Buffey, A. J., M. P. Herring, C. K. Langley, A. E. Donnelly, and B. P. Carson. 2022. "The Acute Effects of Interrupting Prolonged Sitting Time in Adults with Standing and Light-Intensity Walking on Biomarkers of Cardiometabolic Health in Adults: A Systematic Review and Meta-analysis." *Sports Medicine* 52(8): 1765–1787.

Carson, J. A. S., A. H. Lichtenstein, C. A. M. Anderson, L. J. Appel, P. M. Kris-Etherton, K. A. Meyer, K. Petersen, T. Polonsky, and L. Van Horn. 2020. "Dietary Cholesterol and Cardiovascular Risk: A Science Advisory from the American Heart Association." *Circulation* 141(3): e39–e53.

Centers for Disease Control and Prevention (CDC). 2015. "Work Organization Characteristics (NHIS 2015) Charts." CDC. Last updated November 2020. https://wwwn.cdc.gov/NIOSH-WHC/chart/ohs-workorg?OU=*&T=OU&V=R.

———. 2023. "Your Diabetes Care Schedule." CDC, December 19. https://www.cdc.gov/diabetes/treatment/your-diabetes-care-schedule.html.

———. 2024. "National Diabetes Statistics Report." CDC, May 15. https://www.cdc.gov/diabetes/php/data-research.

Ceriello, A., G. Lucisano, F. Prattichizzo, B. Eliasson, S. Franzén, A.-M. Svensson, and A. Nicolucci. 2021. "Variability in Body Weight and the Risk of Cardiovascular Complications in Type 2 Diabetes: Results from the Swedish National Diabetes Register." *Cardiovascular Diabetology* 20(1): 173.

Chastain, R. 2013. "What to Say at the Doctor's Office." *Dances with Fat* (blog), April 1. https://danceswithfat.org/2013/04/01/what-to-say-at-the-doctors-office.

Chatterjee, R., C. A. Davenport, L. P. Svetkey, B. C. Batch, P.-H. Lin, V. S. Ramachandran, et al. 2017. "Serum Potassium Is a Predictor of Incident Diabetes in African Americans with Normal Aldosterone: The Jackson Heart Study." *The American Journal of Clinical Nutrition* 105(2): 442–449.

Chen, C., J. Liu, M. Sun, W. Liu, J. Han, and H. Wang. 2019. "Acupuncture for Type 2 Diabetes Mellitus: A Systematic Review and Meta-Analysis of Randomized Controlled Trials." *Complementary Therapies in Clinical Practice* 36: 100–112.

Chou, H.-W., J.-L. Wang, C.-H. Chang, J.-J. Lee, W.-Y. Shau, and M.-S. Lai. 2013. "Risk of Severe Dysglycemia Among Diabetic Patients Receiving Levofloxacin, Ciprofloxacin, or Moxifloxacin in Taiwan." *Clinical Infectious Diseases* 57(7): 971–980.

Christel, D. A., and S. C. Dunn. 2016. "Average American Women's Clothing Size: Comparing National Health and Nutritional Examination Surveys (1988–2010) to ASTM International Misses & Women's Plus Size Clothing." *International Journal of Fashion Design, Technology and Education* 10(2): 129–136.

Chuengsamarn, S., S. Rattanamongkolgul, R. Luechapudiporn, C. Phisalaphong, and S. Jirawatnotai. 2012. "Curcumin Extract for Prevention of Type 2 Diabetes." *Diabetes Care* 35(11): 2121–2127.

Cleveland Clinic. n.d. "Diaphragmatic Breathing." Last modified March 30, 2022. https://my.clevelandclinic.org/health/articles/9445-diaphragmatic-breathing.

Collins, L., and R. A. Costello. 2024. "Glucagon-Like Peptide-1 Receptor Agonists." *StatPearls*. Updated February 29, 2024. https://www.ncbi.nlm.nih.gov/books/NBK551568.

ConsumerLab.com. n.d. "About ConsumerLab.com." Accessed August 16, 2024. https://www.consumerlab.com/about.

Cook-Cottone, C. P. 2015. *Mindfulness and Yoga for Embodied Self-Regulation: A Primer for Mental Health Professionals.* New York: Springer.

Courtney, J. 2008. "Size Acceptance as a Grief Process: Observations from Psychotherapy with Lesbian Feminists." *Journal of Lesbian Studies* 12(4): 347–363.

Crandall, J. P., K. Mather, S. N. Rajpathak, R. Goldberg, K. Watson, S. Foo, R. Ratner, E. Barrett-Connor, and M. Temprosa, on behalf of the Diabetes Prevention Program (DPP) Research Group. 2017. "Statin Use and Risk of Developing Diabetes: Results from the Diabetes Prevention Program." *BMJ Open Diabetes Research and Care* 5: e000438.

Crawford, C., B. Avula, A. T. Lindsey, A. Walter, K. Katragunta, I. A. Khan, and P. Deuster. 2022. "Analysis of Select Dietary Supplement Products Marketed to Support or Boost the Immune System." *JAMA Network Open* 5(8): e2226040.

Crowley, J., L. Ball, and G. J. Hiddink. 2019. "Nutrition in Medical Education: A Systematic Review." *Lancet Planetary Health* 3(9): e379–e389.

Darby, R., N. E. Henniger, and C. R. Harris. 2014. "Reactions to Physician-Inspired Shame and Guilt." *Basic and Applied Social Psychology* 36(1): 9–26.

Defronzo, R. A. 2009. "From the Triumvirate to the Ominous Octet: A New Paradigm for the Treatment of Type 2 Diabetes Mellitus." *Diabetes* 58(4): 773–795.

Dennick, K., J. Sturt, D. Hessler, E. Purssell, B. Hunter, J. Oliver, and L. Fisher. 2015. "High Rates of Elevated Diabetes Distress in Research Populations: A Systematic Review and Meta-Analysis." *International Diabetes Nursing* 12(3): 93–107.

Deyno, S., K. Eneyew, S. Seyfe, N. Tuyiringire, E. L. Peter, R. A. Muluye, C. U. Tolo, and P. E. Ogwang. 2019. "Efficacy and Safety of Cinnamon in Type 2 Diabetes Mellitus and Pre-Diabetes Patients: A Meta-Analysis and Meta-Regression." *Diabetes Research and Clinical Practice* 156: 107815.

Dick, W. R., E. A. Fletcher, and S. A. Shah. 2016. "Reduction of Fasting Blood Glucose and Hemoglobin A1c Using Oral Aloe Vera: A Meta-Analysis." *Journal of Alternative and Complementary Medicine* 22(6): 450–457.

Dong, H., N. Wang, L. Zhao, and F. Lu. 2012. "Berberine in the Treatment of Type 2 Diabetes Mellitus: A Systematic Review and Meta-Analysis." *Evidence Based Complementary and Alternative Medicine* 2012: 591654.

Dong, J.-Y., P. Xun, K. He, and L.-Q. Qin. 2011. "Magnesium Intake and Risk of Type 2 Diabetes: Meta-Analysis of Prospective Cohort Studies." *Diabetes Care* 34(9): 2116–2122.

Dubey, P., V. Thakur, and M. Chattopadhyay. 2020. "Role of Minerals and Trace Elements in Diabetes and Insulin Resistance." *Nutrients* 12(6): 1864.

Dusenbery, M. 2018. "Doctors Told Her She Was Just Fat. She Actually Had Cancer." *Cosmopolitan,* April 17. https://www.cosmopolitan.com/health-fitness/a19608429 /medical-fatshaming.

Duvivier, B. M. F. M., N. C. Schaper, M. K. C. Hesselink, L. van Kan, N. Stienen, B. Winkens, A. Koster, and H. H. C. M. Savelberg. 2017. "Breaking Sitting with Light Activities vs Structured Exercise: A Randomised Crossover Study Demonstrating Benefits for Glycaemic Control and Insulin Sensitivity in Type 2 Diabetes." *Diabetologia* 60(3): 490–498.

Ekmekcioglu, C., D. Haluza, and M. Kundi. 2017. "25-Hydroxyvitamin D Status and Risk for Colorectal Cancer and Type 2 Diabetes Mellitus: A Systematic Review and Meta-Analysis of Epidemiological Studies." *International Journal of Environmental Research and Public Health* 14(2): 127.

Ellis, R. R. 2023. "They Lost Weight on Wegovy—The Same Drug as Ozempic. Here's What Happened When They Stopped Taking It." *Fortune,* March 14. https:// fortune.com/well/2023/03/14/ozempic-wegovy-what-happens-when-you-stop-taking.

Epstein, L. H., J. L. Temple, J. N. Roemmich, and M. E. Bouton. 2009. "Habituation as a Determinant of Human Food Intake." *Psychological Review* 116(2): 384–407.

Ernst, M. M., and L. H. Epstein. 2002. "Habituation of Responding for Food in Humans." *Appetite* 38(3): 224–234.

Fang, X., H. Han, M. Li, C. Liang, Z. Fan, J. Aaseth, J. He, S. Montgomery, and Y. Cao. 2016. "Dose-Response Relationship Between Dietary Magnesium Intake and Risk of Type 2 Diabetes Mellitus: A Systematic Review and Meta-Regression Analysis of Prospective Cohort Studies." *Nutrients* 8(11): 739.

Fang, X., K. Wang, D. Han, X. He, J. Wei, L. Zhao, et al. 2016. "Dietary Magnesium Intake and the Risk of Cardiovascular Disease, Type 2 Diabetes, and All-Cause Mortality: A Dose–Response Meta-Analysis of Prospective Cohort Studies." *BMC Medicine* 14(1): 210.

Felton, R. 2021. "Beware Dietary Supplements Marketed Online." *Consumer Reports,* March 9. https://www.consumerreports.org/health/beware-dietary-supplements -marketed-online-a6110635129.

Ferrari, M., M. Dal Cin, and M. Steele. 2017. "Self-Compassion Is Associated with Optimum Self-Care Behaviour, Medical Outcomes and Psychological Well-Being in a Cross-Sectional Sample of Adults with Diabetes." *Diabetic Medicine* 34(11): 1546–1553.

Field, A. E., J. E. Manson, C. B. Taylor, W. C. Willett, and G. A. Colditz. 2004. "Association of Weight Change, Weight Control Practices, and Weight Cycling Among Women in the Nurses' Health Study II." *International Journal of Obesity and Related Metabolic Disorders* 28(9): 1134–1142.

Fiskin, G., and N. Sahin. 2021. "Nonpharmacological Management of Gestational Diabetes Mellitus: Diaphragmatic Breathing Exercise." *Alternative Therapies in Health and Medicine* 27(S1): 90–96.

Flegal, K. M., B. I. Graubard, D. F. Williamson, and M. H. Gail. 2005. "Excess Deaths Associated with Underweight, Overweight, and Obesity." *Journal of the American Medical Association* 293(15): 1861–1867.

Francois, M. E., J. C. Baldi, P. J. Manning, S. J. E. Lucas, J. A. Hawley, M. J. A. Williams, and J. D. Cotter. 2014. "'Exercise Snacks' Before Meals: A Novel Strategy to Improve Glycaemic Control in Individuals with Insulin Resistance." *Diabetologia* 57(7): 1437–1445.

French, R. 2023. "Supplement Brands, Amazon and FDA Weigh in on Counterfeit Products." *Natural Products Insider*, August 16. https://www.naturalproductsinsider .com/supplement-regulations/supplement-brands-amazon-and-fda-weigh-in-on -counterfeit-products-.

Future Market Insights. 2023. "Dietary Supplements Market Is Expected to Grow US$ 163.66 Billion by 2033." *Yahoo! Finance*, November 14. https://finance.yahoo .com/news/dietary-supplements-market-expected-grow-130000664.html.

Gahche, J. J., R. L. Bailey, N. Potischman, A. G. Ershow, K. A. Herrick, N. Ahluwalia, and J. T. Dwyer. 2018. "Federal Monitoring of Dietary Supplement Use in the Resident, Civilian, Noninstitutionalized US Population, National Health and Nutrition Examination Survey." *Journal of Nutrition* 148(Suppl 2): 1436S–1444S.

Gao, Y., Q.-Y. Li, T. Finni, and A. J. Pesola. 2024. "Enhanced Muscle Activity During Interrupted Sitting Improves Glycemic Control in Overweight and Obese Men." *Scandinavian Journal of Medicine and Science in Sports* 34(4): e14628.

Garrow, D., and L. E. Egede. 2006. "Association Between Complementary and Alternative Medicine Use, Preventive Care Practices, and Use of Conventional Medical Services Among Adults with Diabetes." *Diabetes Care* 29(1): 15–9.

Goldie, C., A. J. Taylor, P. Nguyen, C. McCoy, X.-Q. Zhao, and D. Preiss. 2016. "Niacin Therapy and the Risk of New-Onset Diabetes: A Meta-Analysis of Randomised Controlled Trials." *Heart* 102(3): 198–203.

Gong, J., K. Fang, H. Dong, D. Wang, M. Hu, and F. Lu. 2016. "Effect of Fenugreek on Hyperglycaemia and Hyperlipidemia in Diabetes and Prediabetes: A Meta-Analysis." *Journal of Ethnopharmacology* 194: 260–268.

Gonzalez, J. S., L. Fisher, and W. H. Polonsky. 2011. "Depression in Diabetes: Have We Been Missing Something Important?" *Diabetes Care* 34(1): 236–239. Erratum in: *Diabetes Care* 34(11): 2488.

Gordon, A. 2020. *What We Don't Talk About When We Talk About Fat.* Boston: Beacon Press.

Griffen, T. C., E. Naumann, and T. Hildebrandt. 2018. "Mirror Exposure Therapy for Body Image Disturbances and Eating Disorders: A Review." *Clinical Psychology Review* 65: 163–174.

Harding, A.-H., N. J. Wareham, S. A. Bingham, K. Khaw, R. Luben, A. Welch, and N. G. Forouhi. 2008. "Plasma Vitamin C Level, Fruit and Vegetable Consumption, and the Risk of New-Onset Type 2 Diabetes Mellitus: The European Prospective

Investigation of Cancer–Norfolk Prospective Study." *Archives of Internal Medicine* 168(14): 1493–1499.

Harrison, C. 2019. *Anti-Diet: Reclaim Your Time, Money, Well-Being, and Happiness Through Intuitive Eating.* New York: Little, Brown Spark.

Hassani, S. S., F. F. Arezodar, S. S. Esmaeili, and M. Gholami-Fesharaki. 2019. "Effect of Fenugreek Use on Fasting Blood Glucose, Glycosylated Hemoglobin, Body Mass Index, Waist Circumference, Blood Pressure and Quality of Life in Patients with Type 2 Diabetes Mellitus: A Randomized, Double-Blinded, Placebo-Controlled Clinical Trials." *Galen Medical Journal* 30(8): e1432.

Hegde, S. V., P. Adhikari, N. K. Subbalakshmi, M. Nandini, G. M. Rao, and V. D'Souza. 2012. "Diaphragmatic Breathing Exercise as a Therapeutic Intervention for Control of Oxidative Stress in Type 2 Diabetes Mellitus." *Complementary Therapies in Clinical Practice* 18(3): 151–153.

Helleputte, S., J. E. Yardley, S. N. Scott, J. Stautemas, L. Jansseune, J. Marlier, T. De Backer, B. Lapauw, and P. Calders. 2023. "Effects of Postprandial Exercise on Blood Glucose Levels in Adults with Type 1 Diabetes: A Review." *Diabetologia* 66(7): 1179–1191.

Herzog Ramos, M., J. M. Silva, T. A. Venturini De Oliveira, J. da Silva Batista, M. Cattafesta, L. Bresciani Salaroli, and F. L. Pires Soares. 2022. "Intuitive Eating and Body Appreciation in Type 2 Diabetes." *Journal of Health Psychology* 27(2): 255–267.

Himmelstein, M. S., A. C. Incollingo Belsky, and A. J. Tomiyama. 2014. "The Weight of Stigma: Cortisol Reactivity to Manipulated Weight Stigma." *Obesity* 23(2): 368–374.

Hinault, C., P. Caroli-Bosc, F. Bost, and N. Chevalier. 2023. "Critical Overview on Endocrine Disruptors in Diabetes Mellitus." *International Journal of Molecular Sciences* 24(5): 4537.

Hsieh, R.-Y., I.-C. Huang, C. Chen, and J.-Y. Sung. 2023. "Effects of Oral Alpha-Lipoic Acid Treatment on Diabetic Polyneuropathy: A Meta-Analysis and Systematic Review." *Nutrients* 15(16): 3634.

Huseini, H. F., B. Larijani, R. Heshmat, H. Fakhrzadeh, B. Radjabipour, T. Toliat, and M. Raza. 2006. "The Efficacy of Silybum Marianum (L.) Gaertn. (Silymarin) in the Treatment of Type II Diabetes: A Randomized, Double-Blind, Placebo-Controlled, Clinical Trial." *Phytotherapy Research* 20(12): 1036–1039.

Hussain, S. M., A. B. Newman, L. J. Beilin, A. M. Tonkin, R. L. Woods, J. T. Neumann, et al. 2023. "Associations of Change in Body Size with All-Cause and Cause-Specific Mortality Among Healthy Older Adults." *JAMA Network Open* 6(4): e237482.

Hwang, J. L., and R. E. Weiss. 2014. "Steroid-Induced Diabetes: a Clinical and Molecular Approach to Understanding and Treatment." *Diabetes Metabolism Research and Reviews* 30(2): 96–102.

Iizuka, K. 2022. "Is the Use of Artificial Sweeteners Beneficial for Patients with Diabetes Mellitus? The Advantages and Disadvantages of Artificial Sweeteners." *Nutrients* 14(21): 4446.

Innes, K. E., and T. K. Selfe. 2016. "Yoga for Adults with Type 2 Diabetes: A Systematic Review of Controlled Trials." *Journal of Diabetes Research* 2016: 6979370.

International Diabetes Federation (IDF). 2021. *IDF Diabetes Atlas*, 10th ed. Brussels, Belgium: International Diabetes Federation. https://diabetesatlas.org/atlas/tenth-edition.

Izgu, N., Z. G. Metin, C. Karadas, L. Ozdemir, N. Metinarikan, and D. Corapcioglu. 2020. "Progressive Muscle Relaxation and Mindfulness Meditation on Neuropathic Pain, Fatigue, and Quality of Life in Patients with Type 2 Diabetes: A Randomized Clinical Trial." *Journal of Nursing Scholarship* 52(5): 476–487.

Keys, A., F. Fidanza, M. J. Karvonen, N. Kimura, and H. L. Taylor. 1972. "Indices of Relative Weight and Obesity." *Journal of Chronic Diseases* 25(6): 329–343.

Kokoszka, A., A. Pacura, B. Kostecka, C. E. Lloyd, and N. Sartorius. 2022. "Body Self-Esteem Is Related to Subjective Well-Being, Severity of Depressive Symptoms, BMI, Glycated Hemoglobin Levels, and Diabetes-Related Distress in Type 2 Diabetes." *PLoS One* 17(2): e0263766.

Kolb, L. 2021. "An Effective Model of Diabetes Care and Education: The ADCES7 Self-Care Behaviors." *The Science of Diabetes Self-Management and Care* 47(1): 30–53.

Korkeila, M., A. Rissanen, J. Kaprio, T. I. Sorensen, and M. Koskenvuo. 1999. "Weight-Loss Attempts and Risk of Major Weight Gain: A Prospective Study in Finnish Adults." *American Journal of Clinical Nutrition* 70(6): 965–975.

Køster-Rasmussen, R., M. K. Simonsen, V. Siersma, J. E. Henriksen, B. L. Heitmann, and N. de Fine Olivarius. 2016. "Intentional Weight Loss and Longevity in Overweight Patients with Type 2 Diabetes: A Population-Based Cohort Study." *PLoS ONE* 11(1): e0146889.

Kübler-Ross, E. 2009. *On Death and Dying: What the Dying Have to Teach Doctors, Nurses, Clergy and Their Own Families*, 40th anniversary ed. London: Routledge.

Leproult, R., U. Holmback, and E. Van Cauter. 2014. "Circadian Misalignment Augments Markers of Insulin Resistance and Inflammation, Independently of Sleep Loss." *Diabetes* 63(6): 1860–1869.

Lips, P., M. Eekhoff, N. van Schoor, M. Oosterwerff, R. de Jongh, Y. Krul-Poel, and S. Simsek. 2017. "Vitamin D and Type 2 Diabetes." *Journal of Steroid Biochemistry and Molecular Biology* 173: 280–285.

Lissner, L., P. M. Odell, R. B. D'Agostino, J. Stokes III, B. E. Kreger, A. J. Belanger, and K. D. Brownell. 1991. "Variability of Body Weight and Health Outcomes in the Framingham Population." *New England Journal of Medicine* 324(26): 1839–1844.

Look AHEAD Research Group. 2013. "Cardiovascular Effects of Intensive Lifestyle Intervention in Type 2 Diabetes." *New England Journal of Medicine* 369(2): 145–154. Erratum in: *New England Journal of Medicine* 370(19): 1866.

Majeed-Ariss, R., C. Jackson, P. Knapp, and F. M. Cheater. 2015. "A Systematic Review of Research into Black and Ethnic Minority Patients' Views on Self-Management of Type 2 Diabetes." *Health Expectations* 18(5): 625–642.

Mandel, S. E., B. A. Davis, and M. Secic. 2013. "Effects of Music Therapy and Music-Assisted Relaxation and Imagery on Health-Related Outcomes in Diabetes Education: A Feasibility Study." *Diabetes Educator* 39(4): 568-81.

Marino, R., and M. Misra. 2019. "Extra-Skeletal Effects of Vitamin D." *Nutrients* 11(7): 1460.

Marton, L. T., L. M. Pescinini-e-Salzedas, M. E. Côrtes Camargo, S. M. Barbalho, J. F. dos Santos Haber, R. Vargas Sinatora, C. R. Penteado Detregiachi, R. J. S. Girio, D. Vieira Buchaim, and P. Cincotto dos Santos Bueno. 2021. "The Effects of Curcumin on Diabetes Mellitus: A Systematic Review." *Frontiers in Endocrinology* 12: 669448.

McKennon, S. A. 2000. "Non-Pharmaceutical Intervention Options for Type 2 Diabetes: Complementary Health Approaches and Integrative Health (Including Natural Products and Mind/Body Practices)." In *Endotext*, edited by K. R. Feingold, B. Anawalt, M. R. Blackman, A. Boyce, G. Chrousos, et al. South Dartmouth, MA: MDText.com.

Mensinger, J. L., T. L. Tylka, and M. E. Calamari. 2018. "Mechanisms Underlying Weight Status and Health Care Avoidance in Women: A Study of Weight Stigma, Body-Related Shame and Guilt, and Health Care Stress." *Body Image* 25: 139–147.

Millard, E. 2023. "How Nutrition Education for Doctors Is Evolving." *Time*, May 24. https://time.com/6282404/nutrition-education-doctors.

Mudaliar, S. 2023. "The Evolution of Diabetes Treatment Through the Ages: From Starvation Diets to Insulin, Incretins, SGLT2-Inhibitors and Beyond." *Journal of the Indian Institute of Science* 103: 123–133.

Nam, G. E., W. Kim, K. Han, C.-W. Lee, Y. Kwon, B. Han, et al. 2020. "Body Weight Variability and the Risk of Cardiovascular Outcomes and Mortality in Patients with Type 2 Diabetes: A Nationwide Cohort Study." *Diabetes Care* 43(9): 2234–2241.

National Institute of Diabetes and Digestive and Kidney Diseases (NIDDK). "The A1C Test & Diabetes." NIDDK.com. Last reviewed April 2018. https://www.niddk.nih.gov/health-information/diagnostic-tests/a1c-test.

National Institutes of Health (NIH). 2022. "Chromium: Fact Sheet for Health Professionals." Last updated June 2, 2022. https://ods.od.nih.gov/factsheets/Chromium-HealthProfessional.

Neelakantan, N., M. Narayanan, R. J. de Souza, and R. M. van Dam. 2014. "Effect of Fenugreek (Trigonella foenum-graecum L.) Intake on Glycemia: A Meta-Analysis of Clinical Trials." *Nutrition Journal* 13: 7.

NIH Technology Assessment Conference Panel. 1993. "Methods for Voluntary Weight Loss and Control." *Annals of Internal Medicine* 119: 764–770.

Noble, M. n.d. "Body Acceptance Begins with Grieving the Thin Ideal." *Meredith Noble* (blog). Accessed March 28, 2024. https://www.meredithnoble.com/blog/body-acceptance-begins-with-grieving-the-thin-ideal.

Nummenmaa, L., R. Hari, J. K. Hietanen, and E. Glerean. 2018. "Maps of Subjective Feelings." *Proceedings of the National Academy of Sciences* 115(37): 9198–9203.

O'Hara, L., and J. Taylor. 2018. "What's Wrong with the 'War on Obesity'? A Narrative Review of the Weight-Centered Health Paradigm and Development of the 3C Framework to Build Critical Competency for a Paradigm Shift." *SAGE Open* 8(2).

Oliver, J. E. 2006. *Fat Politics: The Real Story behind America's Obesity Epidemic.* New York: Oxford University Press.

Otten, J. J., J. P. Hellwig, and L. D. Meyers, eds. 2006. *Dietary Reference Intakes: The Essential Guide to Nutrient Requirements.* Washington, DC: National Academies Press, Institute of Medicine.

Pan, A., E. S. Schernhammer, Q. Sun, and F. B. Hu. 2011. "Rotating Night Shift Work and Risk of Type 2 Diabetes: Two Prospective Cohort Studies in Women." *PLoS Medicine* 8(12): e1001141.

Park, K.-Y., H.-S. Hwang, K.-H. Cho, K. Han, G. E. Nam, Y. H. Kim, Y. Kwon, and Y.-G. Park. 2019. "Body Weight Fluctuation as a Risk Factor for Type 2 Diabetes: Results from a Nationwide Cohort Study." *Journal of Clinical Medicine* 8(7): 950.

Parker, E. D., J. Lin, T. Mahoney, N. Ume, G. Yang, R. A. Gabbay, N. A. ElSayed, and R. R. Bannuru. 2024. "Economic Costs of Diabetes in the US in 2022." *Diabetes Care* 47(1): 26–43.

Pearl, R. L., T. A. Wadden, C. M. Hopkins, J. A. Shaw, M. R. Hayes, Z. M. Bakizada, et al. 2017. "Association Between Weight Bias Internalization and Metabolic Syndrome Among Treatment-Seeking Individuals with Obesity." *Obesity* 25(2): 317–322.

Pelczyńska, M., M. Moszak, and P. Bogdański. 2022. "The Role of Magnesium in the Pathogenesis of Metabolic Disorders." *Nutrients* 14(9): 1714.

Piller, C. 2019. "The War on 'Prediabetes' Could Be a Boon for Pharma—But Is It Good Medicine?" *Science*, March 7. https://www.science.org/content/article/war -prediabetes-could-be-boon-pharma-it-good-medicine.

Pires Soares, F. L., M. H. Ramos, M. Gramelisch, R. de Paula Pego Silva, J. da Silva Batista, M. Cattafesta, and L. B. Salaroli. 2021. "Intuitive Eating Is Associated with Glycemic Control in Type 2 Diabetes." *Eating and Weight Disorders* 26(2): 599–608.

Polivy, J., and C. P. Herman. 1980. "Experimental and Clinical Aspects of Restrained Eating." In *Obesity: Basic Mechanisms and Treatment*, edited by A. J. Strunkard, 208–225. Philadelphia: W. B. Saunders.

Pollack, A. 2013. "AMA Recognizes Obesity as a Disease." *New York Times*, June 18. https://www.nytimes.com/2013/06/19/business/ama-recognizes-obesity-as-a-disease .html.

Potter, L., K. Wallston, P. Trief, J. Ulbrecht, V. Juth, and J. Smyth. 2015. "Attributing Discrimination to Weight: Associations with Well-Being, Self-Care, and Disease Status in patients with Type 2 Diabetes Mellitus." *Journal of Behavioral Medicine* 38(6): 863–875.

Priya, G., and S. Kalra. 2018. "Mind-Body Interactions and Mindfulness Meditation in Diabetes." *European Endocrinology* 14(1): 35–41.

Proschaska, J. O., and C. C. DiClemente. 1983. "Stages and Processes of Self-Change of Smoking: Toward an Integrative Model of Change." *Journal of Consulting and Clinical Psychology* 51(3): 390–395.

Puhl, R. M., and K. D. Brownell. 2006. "Confronting and Coping with Weight Stigma: An Investigation of Overweight and Obese Adults." *Obesity* 14(10): 1802–1815.

Quansah, D. Y., J. Gross, L. Gilbert, C. Helbling, A. Horsch, and J. J. Puder. 2019. "Intuitive Eating Is Associated with Weight and Glucose Control During Pregnancy and in the Early Postpartum Period in Women with Gestational Diabetes Mellitus: A Clinical Cohort Study." *Eating Behaviors* 34: 101304.

Quansah, D. Y., L. Gilbert, J. Gross, A. Horsch, and J. J. Puder. 2021. "Intuitive Eating Is Associated with Improved Health Indicators at 1-Year Postpartum in Women with Gestational Diabetes Mellitus." *Journal of Health Psychology* 26(8): 1168–1184.

Quansah, D. Y., S. Schenk, L. Gilbert, A. Arhab, J. Gross, P.-M. Marques-Vidal, E. G. Rodriguez, D. Hans, A. Horsch, and J. J. Puder. 2022. "Intuitive Eating Behavior, Diet Quality and Metabolic Health in the Postpartum in Women with Gestational Diabetes." *Nutrients* 14(20): 4272.

Quittkat, H. L., A. S. Hartmann, R. Düsing, U. Buhlmann, and S. Vocks. 2019. "Body Dissatisfaction, Importance of Appearance, and Body Appreciation in Men and Women Over the Lifespan." *Frontiers in Psychiatry.*10: 864.

Reutrakul, S., and B. Mokhlesi. 2017. "Obstructive Sleep Apnea and Diabetes: A State of the Art Review." *Chest* 152(5): 1070–1086.

Rhee, E.-J., J.-H. Cho, H. Kwon, S. E. Park, C.-Y. Park, K.-W. Oh, S.-W. Park, and W.-Y. Lee. 2018. "Increased Risk of Diabetes Development in Individuals with Weight Cycling Over 4 Years: The Kangbuk Samsung Health Study." *Diabetes Research and Clinical Practice* 139: 230–238.

Richter, B., B. Hemmingsen, M.-I. Metzendorf, and Y. Takwoingi. 2018. "Development of Type 2 Diabetes Mellitus in People with Intermediate Hyperglycaemia." *Cochrane Database of Systematic Reviews* 10: CD012661.

Rios-Leyvraz, M., and J. Montez. 2022. *Health Effects of the Use of Non-Sugar Sweeteners: A Systematic Review and Meta-Analysis.* Geneva: World Health Organization. https://www.who.int/publications/i/item/9789240046429.

Rzehak, P., C. Meisinger, G. Woelke, S. Brasche, G. Strube, and J. Heinrich. 2007. "Weight Change, Weight Cycling and Mortality in the ERFORT Male Cohort Study." *European Journal of Epidemiology* 22(10): 665–673.

Sandham, C., and E. Deacon. 2023. "The Role of Self-Compassion in Diabetes Management: A Rapid Review." *Frontiers in Psychology* 14: 1123157.

Scheiner, G. 2020. *Think Like a Pancreas: A Practical Guide to Managing Diabetes with Insulin.* New York: Hachette Go.

Schneider, E. C., A. Shah, M. M. Doty, R. Tikkanen, K. Fields, and R. D. Williams II. 2021. "Mirror, Mirror 2021: Reflecting Poorly: Health Care in the U.S. Compared

to Other High-Income Countries." *Commonwealth Fund*, August 4. https://www
.commonwealthfund.org/publications/fund-reports/2021/aug/mirror-mirror-2021
-reflecting-poorly.

Shah, M., C. Vasandani, B. Adams-Huet, and A. Garg. 2018. "Comparison of Nutrient
Intakes in South Asians with Type 2 Diabetes Mellitus and Controls Living in the
United States." *Diabetes Research and Clinical Practice* 138: 47–56.

Shan, Z., H. Ma, M. Xie, P. Yan, Y. Guo, W. Bao, Y. Rong, C. L. Jackson, F. B. Hu,
and L. Liu. 2015. "Sleep Duration and Risk of Type 2 Diabetes: A Meta-Analysis
of Prospective Studies." *Diabetes Care* 38(3): 529–537.

Shane-McWhorter, L. 2013. "Dietary Supplements for Diabetes Are Decidedly Popular:
Help Your Patients Decide." *Diabetes Spectrum* 26(4): 259–266.

Siegel, D. J. 2010. *Mindsight: The New Science of Personal Transformation*. New York:
Bantam Books.

Smink, F. R. E., D. van Hoeken, and H. W. Hoek. 2012. "Epidemiology of Eating
Disorders: Incidence, Prevalence and Mortality Rates." *Current Psychiatry Reports*
14(4): 406–414.

Stoddard, J. A., and N. Afari. 2014. *The Big Book of ACT Metaphors: A Practitioner's
Guide to Experiential Exercises and Metaphors in Acceptance and Commitment
Therapy*. Oakland, CA: New Harbinger Publications.

Strom, J. L., and L. E. Egede. 2012. "The Impact of Social Support on Outcomes in
Adult Patients with Type 2 Diabetes: A Systematic Review." *Current Diabetes
Reports* 12(6): 769–781.

Stunkard, A., and M. McClaren-Hume. 1959. "The Results of Treatment for Obesity:
A Review of the Literature and Report of a Series." AMA *Archives of Internal
Medicine* 103(1): 79–85.

Suez, J., T. Korem, D. Zeevi, G. Zilberman-Schapira, C.A. Thaiss, O. Maza, et al.
2014. "Artificial Sweeteners Induce Glucose Intolerance by Altering the Gut
Microbiota." *Nature* 514: 181–186.

Suksomboon, N., N. Poolsup, and A. Yuwanakorn. 2014. "Systematic Review and
Meta-Analysis of the Efficacy and Safety of Chromium Supplementation in
Diabetes." *Journal of Clinical Pharmacy and Therapeutics* 39(3): 292–306.

Swithers, S. E., and W. G. Hall. 1994. "Does Oral Experience Terminate Ingestion?"
Appetite 23(2): 113–138.

Tai-Seale, M., T. G. McGuire, and W. Zhang. 2007. "Time Allocation in Primary
Care Office Visits." *Health Services Research* 42(5): 1871–1894.

Tanenbaum, M. L., R. N. Adams, J. S. Gonzalez, S. J. Hanes, and K. K. Hood. 2018.
"Adapting and Validating a Measure of Diabetes-Specific Self-Compassion."
Journal of Diabetes and Its Complications 32(2): 196–202.

Tribole, E., and E. Resch. 2020. *Intuitive Eating: A Revolutionary Anti-Diet Approach*,
4th ed. New York: St. Martin's Essentials.

Tylka, T. L. 2006. "Development and Psychometric Evaluation of a Measure of Intuitive Eating." *Journal of Counseling Psychology* 53(2): 226–240.

Tylka, T. L., R. A. Annunziato, D. Burgard, S. Daníelsdóttir, E. Shuman, C. Davis, and R. M. Calogero. 2014. "The Weight-Inclusive Versus Weight-Normative Approach to Health: Evaluating the Evidence for Prioritizing Well-Being over Weight Loss." *Journal of Obesity* 2014: 983495.

Tylka, T. L., R. M. Calogero, and S. Daníelsdóttir. 2019. "Intuitive Eating Is Connected to Self-Reported Weight Stability in Community Women and Men." *Eating Disorders* 28(3): 256–264.

Tylka, T. L., and A. M. Kroon Van Diest. 2013. "The Intuitive Eating Scale–2: Item Refinement and Psychometric Evaluation with College Women and Men." *Journal of Counseling Psychology* 60(1): 137–153.

Tylka, T. L., C. Maïano, M. Fuller-Tyszkiewicz, J. Linardon, C. B. Burnette, J. Todd, and V. Swami. 2024. "The Intuitive Eating Scale-3: Development and Psychometric Evaluation." *Appetite* 199: 107407.

US Department of Agriculture (USDA). 2024. "Summary Findings: Food Price Outlook, 2024 and 2025." Updated July 25, 2024. https://www.ers.usda.gov/data-products/food -price-outlook/summary-findings.

US Department of Health and Human Services (HHS), Office of Disease Prevention and Health Promotion. n.d. "Social Determinants of Health." Accessed September 20, 2023. https://health.gov/healthypeople/objectives-and-data/social-determinants -health.

US Food and Drug Administration (FDA). 2022. "FDA 101: Dietary Supplements." Last updated June 2, 2022. https://www.fda.gov/consumers/consumer-updates/fda -101-dietary-supplements.

Vashum, K. P., M. McEvoy, Z. Shi, A. H. Milton, M. R. Islam, D. Sibbritt, A. Patterson, J. Byles, D. Loxton, and J. Attia. 2013. "Is Dietary Zinc Protective for Type 2 Diabetes? Results from the Australian Longitudinal Study on Women's Health." *BMC Endocrine Disorders* 13: 40.

Villegas, R., Y.-T. Gao, Q. Dai, G. Yang, H. Cai, H. Li, W. Zheng, and X. O. Shu. 2009. "Dietary Calcium and Magnesium Intakes and the Risk of Type 2 Diabetes: The Shanghai Women's Health Study." *American Journal of Clinical Nutrition* 89(4): 1059–1067.

Vimalananda, V. G., J. R. Palmer, H. Gerlovin, L. A. Wise, J. L. Rosenzweig, L. Rosenberg, and E. A. Ruiz Narváez. 2015. "Night-Shift Work and Incident Diabetes Among African-American Women." *Diabetologia* 58(4): 699-706.

Wartella, E. A., A. H. Lichtenstein, and C. S. Boon, eds. 2010. "Front-of-Package Nutrition Rating Systems and Symbols: Phase I Report." Washington, DC: National Academies Press, Institute of Medicine (US) Committee on Examination of Front-of-Package Nutrition Rating Systems and Symbols.

Westwater, M. L., P. C. Fletcher, and H. Ziauddeen. 2016. "Sugar Addiction: The State of the Science." *European Journal of Nutrition* 55(Suppl 2): 55–69.

Wheeler, B. J., J. Lawrence, M. Chae, H. Paterson, A. R. Gray, D. Healey, D. M. Reith, and B. J. Taylor. 2016. "Intuitive Eating Is Associated with Glycaemic Control in Adolescents with Type I Diabetes Mellitus." *Appetite* 96: 160–165.

Wilding, J. P. H., R. L. Batterham, M. Davies, L. F. Van Gaal, K. Kandler, K. Konakli, et al. 2022. "Weight Regain and Cardiometabolic Effects After Withdrawal of Semaglutide: The STEP 1 Trial Extension." *Diabetes, Obesity, and Metabolism* 24(8): 1553–1564.

Willig, A. L., B. S. Richardson, A. Agne, and A. Cherrington. 2014. "Intuitive Eating Practices Among African-American Women Living with Type 2 Diabetes: A Qualitative Study." *Journal of the Academy of Nutrition and Dietetics* 114(6): 889–896.

Wirth, M. D., C. E. Blake, J. R. Hébert, X. Sui, and S. N. Blair. 2014. "Chronic Weight Dissatisfaction Predicts Type 2 Diabetes Risk: Aerobic Center Longitudinal Study." *Health Psychology* 33(8): 912–919.

Witusik, A., S. Kaczmarek, and T. Pietras. 2022. "The Role of Music Therapy in the Treatment of Patients with Type 2 Diabetes." *Polski Merkuriusz Lekarski* 50(297): 210–212.

Wood-Barcalow, N. L., T. L. Tylka, and C. L. Augustus-Horvath. 2010. "'But I Like My Body': Positive Body Image Characteristics and a Holistic Model for Young-Adult Women." *Body Image* 7(2): 106–116.

Yadav, A., R. M. Kaushik, and R. Kaushik. 2021. "Effects of Diaphragmatic Breathing and Systematic Relaxation on Depression, Anxiety, Stress, and Glycemic Control in Type 2 Diabetes Mellitus." *International Journal of Yoga Therapy* 31(1): Article 13.

Yang, Q. 2010. "Gain Weight by 'Going Diet?' Artificial Sweeteners and the Neurobiology of Sugar Cravings: Neuroscience 2010." *Yale Journal of Biology and Medicine* 83(2): 101–108.

Yin, J., H. Xing, and J. Ye. 2008. "Efficacy of Berberine in Patients with Type 2 Diabetes Mellitus." *Metabolism* 57(5): 712-7.

Zarezadeh, M., V. Musazadeh, E. Foroumandi, M. Keramati, A. Ostadrahimi, and R. A. Mekary. 2023. "The Effect of Cinnamon Supplementation on Glycemic Control in Patients with Type 2 Diabetes or with Polycystic Ovary Syndrome: An Umbrella Meta-Analysis on Interventional Meta-Analyses." *Diabetology and Metabolic Syndrome* 15: 127.

Zhang, X., K. M. Bullard, E. W. Gregg, G. L. Beckles, D. E. Williams, L. E. Barker, A. L. Albright, and G. Imperatore. 2012. "Access to Health Care and Control of ABCs of Diabetes." *Diabetes Care* 35(7): 1566–1571.

Zhang, Z., Y. Zhang, X. Tao, Y. Wang, B. Rao, and H. Shi. 2023. "Effects of Glucomannan Supplementation on Type II Diabetes Mellitus in Humans: A Meta-Analysis." *Nutrients* 15(3): 601.

Zou, H., P. Yin, L. Liu, L. Duan, P. Li, Y. Yang, W. Li, Q. Zong, and X. Yu. 2021. "Association Between Weight Cycling and Risk of Developing Diabetes in Adults: A Systematic Review and Meta-Analysis." *Journal of Diabetes Investigation* 12(4): 625–632.

Janice Dada, MPH, RDN, is a weight-inclusive registered dietitian with a private practice in Newport Beach, CA. She is a certified Intuitive Eating counselor, certified diabetes care and education specialist (CDCES), and certified eating disorders specialist (CEDS). She is passionate about simplifying and destigmatizing the nutrition- and weight-based discourse around diabetes.

Foreword writer **Elyse Resch, MS, RDN,** is a nutrition therapist specializing in eating disorders, Intuitive Eating, and health at every size. She is coauthor of *Intuitive Eating,* and author of *The Intuitive Eating Workbook for Teens* and *The Intuitive Eating Journal.*

Real change *is* possible

For more than fifty years, New Harbinger has published proven-effective self-help books and pioneering workbooks to help readers of all ages and backgrounds improve mental health and well-being, and achieve lasting personal growth. In addition, our spirituality books offer profound guidance for deepening awareness and cultivating healing, self-discovery, and fulfillment.

Founded by psychologist Matthew McKay and Patrick Fanning, New Harbinger is proud to be an independent, employee-owned company.
Our books reflect our core values of integrity, innovation, commitment, sustainability, compassion, and trust. Written by leaders in the field and recommended by therapists worldwide, New Harbinger books are practical, accessible, and provide real tools for real change.

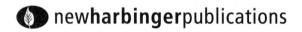 **newharbinger**publications

MORE BOOKS from
NEW HARBINGER PUBLICATIONS

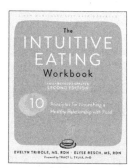
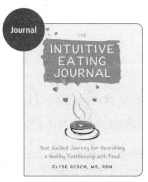
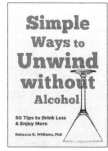
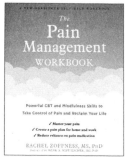
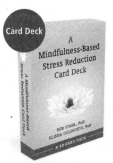
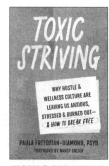

Did you know there are **free tools** you can download for this book?

Free tools are things like **worksheets**, **guided meditation exercises**, and **more** that will help you get the most out of your book.

You can download free tools for this book— whether you bought or borrowed it, in any format, from any source—from the New Harbinger website. All you need is a NewHarbinger.com account. Just use the URL provided in this book to view the free tools that are available for it. Then, click on the "download" button for the free tool you want, and follow the prompts that appear to log in to your NewHarbinger.com account and download the material.

You can also save the free tools for this book to your **Free Tools Library** so you can access them again anytime, just by logging in to your account! Just look for this button on the book's free tools page.

+ Save this to my free tools library

If you need help accessing or downloading free tools, visit **newharbinger.com/faq** or contact us at **customerservice@newharbinger.com**.